Alta Bates Summit Medical Center

A CENTURY OF CARING

A PICTORIAL HISTORY OF
ALTA BATES SUMMIT MEDICAL CENTER

Alta Bates Summit Medical Center
Berkeley and Oakland

Alta Bates Summit Medical Center, Berkeley and Oakland
© 2005 by Alta Bates Summit Medical Center
Published 2005
Printed in China

ISBN 0-9761067-0-1

MARKETING AND COMMUNITY RELATIONS DEPARTMENT CO-EDITORS
Jill Keith Gruen, Carolyn E. Kemp

EDITORIAL ADVISORS

Robert J. Albo, MD, Jan Anderson, Marie Bishop, Mary Brown, Arlene Brosnan, Lillian Cadenasso, Michael J. Cassidy, MD, Linda L. Chew, Leland H. Cohn, MD, Michelle Cox, David L. Cutter, Barbara D'Anneo, Leo Dominguez, William G. Donald, MD, Andrea Edge, RN, James B. Florey, MD, E. Pat Gary, MD, Mickey Goldman, Joyce Gray, RN, Robert M. Greene, MD, Elena Griffing, Frances Hanna, Mary Havis, General K. Hilliard, MD, Roger W. Hoag, MD, Bruce A. Horwitz, MD, Ed Jung, Jerome E. Kaufman, MD, Barbara Kelly, Junaid H. Khan, MD, Warren J. Kirk, Alan Lifshay, MD, Peggy Lipper, Thora Loutfi, Paul L. Ludmer, MD, Stephen A. Lundin, Richards P. Lyon, MD, Patricia W. McLaren, Thomas L. McLaren, Vic Meinke, Robert L. Montgomery, Nobie Onishi, Lloyd C. Patterson, MD, Tammy Peterson, Betsy Rodriguez, Donald A. Shimer, Irene Slavens, Tolbert J. Small, MD, Frank E. Staggers Sr., MD, Vertis R. Thompson, MD, Amy Trask

ARCHIVISTS

J. Norman Dizon (Providence Assistant Archivist), Arlene Erb (Alta Bates Summit Volunteer Association), Mary Ann Furuichi (Alta Bates Summit Volunteer Association), Loretta Greene (Providence Archivist), Peter Schmid (Providence Assistant Archivist, Visual Resources)

CENTENNIAL ADVISORY BOARD

Annalee Allen, Polly Armstrong, Mary Brown, Rachel Bryant, Joseph W. Clift, MD, Michelle Cox, Barbara D'Anneo, Jill K. Gruen, Joseph J. Haraburda, Gloria Harmon, Irene Hegarty, Carolyn E. Kemp, Fran Kidd, Thora Loutfi, Stephen A. Lundin, Robert L. Montgomery, Denise Navellier, RN, Herbert E. Stansbury, Arlene Swinderman, Ann Brekke Yungert, RN

PRODUCED BY DIABLO CUSTOM PUBLISHING
EDITOR Angela Noel
ART DIRECTOR Linda Birch
WRITERS Jackie Krentzman, Angela Noel
CONTRIBUTING WRITERS Thomas Flack, Alison Shapiro
COPY EDITOR Matt Jones
EDITORIAL RESEARCHERS Thomas Flack, Michael Krolak,
David Randall, Alison Shapiro
PHOTO RESEARCHER Thomas Flack
EDITORIAL AND PHOTO ADVISORS Harold Adler, Annalee Allen,
Kathleen DiGiovanni, Tom Edwards, Veronica Lee,
Shannon Reynolds, Sayre Van Young
CREATIVE DIRECTOR David Bergeron
EDITORIAL DIRECTOR Jackie Krentzman
SENIOR PROJECT MANAGER Laura-Lee Love
PREPRESS Phil Brown, Mark Dalton, Pete Sonne
VICE PRESIDENT AND GENERAL MANAGER Jim Offel

This book project was undertaken for historical purposes and benefits the programs and services of Alta Bates Summit Medical Center. Every effort has been made to ensure the accuracy of the information herein, relying in large part on the Medical Center's archives. (Photo captions display available information.) Alta Bates Summit Medical Center, Alta Bates Summit Foundation, and Diablo Custom Publishing editors, designers, writers, and researchers regret any possible errors or omissions.

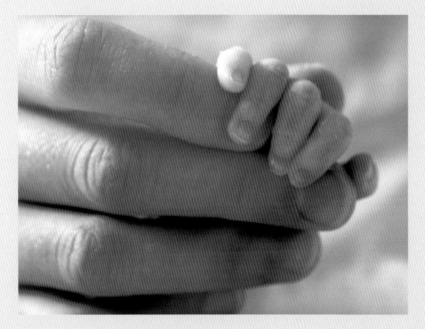

January 2005

THIS BOOK IS DEDICATED to the thousands of men and women who, over the last century, devoted their lives and careers to Alta Bates Summit Medical Center and its five heritage hospitals. For their daily commitment to health care, their communities, and the marvel and mystery of life, we are extremely grateful.

We are honored to have the rare opportunity at this historic moment to collect, discover, and retell the many stories of Alta Bates Summit and our remarkable community.

Warren J. Kirk, President and CEO
Alta Bates Summit Medical Center

Carolyn E. Kemp, Director
Public Relations

Jill Keith Gruen, Administrative Director
Marketing and Community Relations

Stephen A. Lundin, President
Alta Bates Summit Foundation

TABLE OF
contents

 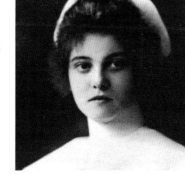
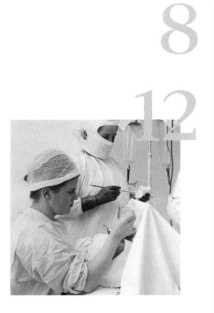

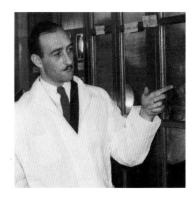

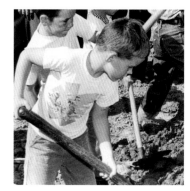

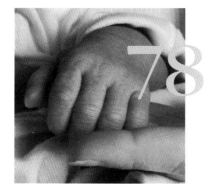
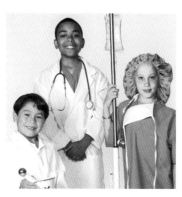

timeless traditions

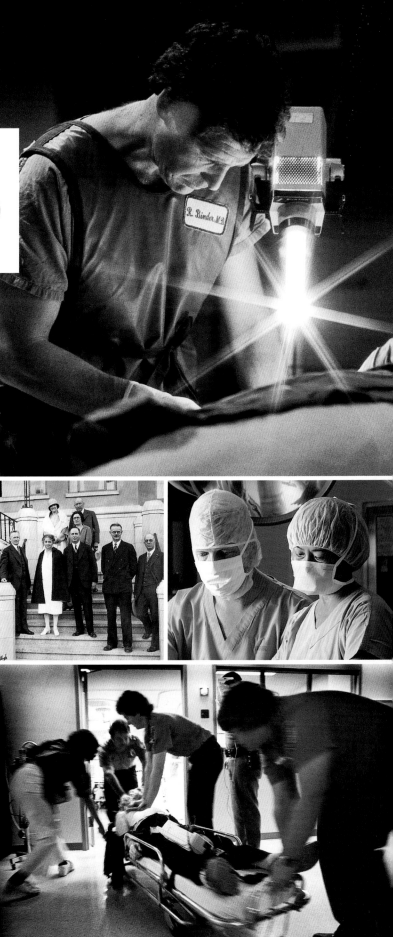

To tell the history of Alta Bates Summit Medical Center is to chronicle a tradition of dedication and service to the East Bay community. Over 100 proud years, five hospitals—Alta Bates, Herrick, Merritt, Peralta, and Providence—would share a mission, make their lasting mark, and become one. Together, they have been a vital resource for health and healing through war and peace, natural catastrophes and man-made discoveries, family crises, local prosperity, and much more.

Certainly, Alta Bates Summit's tradition of dedication is rooted in the unwavering commitment of its founders. The devoted Sisters of Providence, the intrepid, young nurse Alta Alice Miner Bates, the visionary Drs. Samuel Merritt and LeRoy Herrick, and the pioneering Drs. John L. Lohse, W.B. Palamountain, P.N. Jacobson, Hayward G. Thomas and Quinton O. Gilbert of Peralta set a standard of health care excellence that has endured.

Then, as now, the hospitals nurtured innovation and facilitated exceptional performance. Their healing arts have witnessed wondrous advancement: from the turn of the century's introduction to X-ray technology to contemporary computer-aided tomography; from the early, awkward uses of

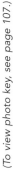

(To view photo key, see page 107.)

8

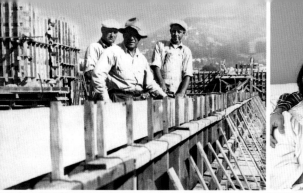
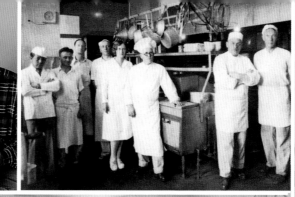
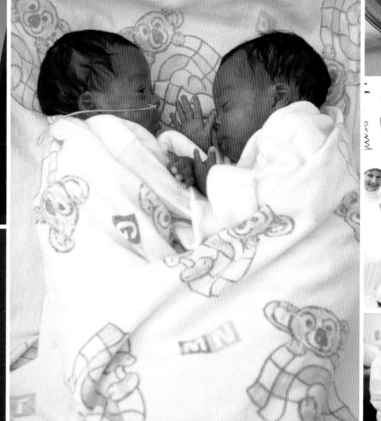
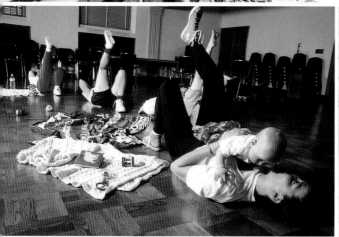
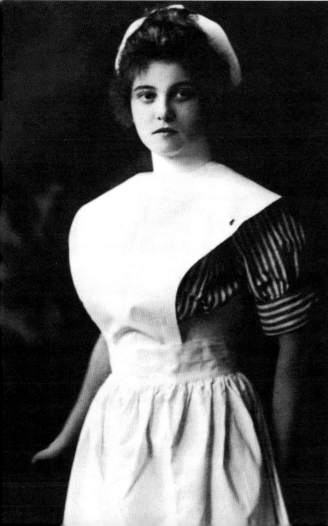
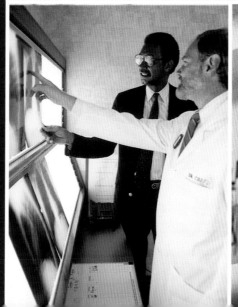
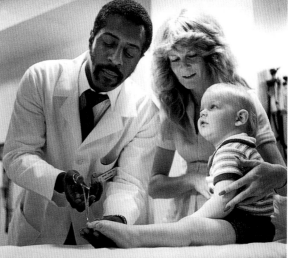

anesthesia to modern open-heart surgery and now minimally invasive procedures and robotics; from an era when home births were popular to the Medical Center's current average of nearly 10,000 babies delivered each year.

Today, Alta Bates Summit Medical Center, with three campuses in Berkeley and Oakland, is the East Bay's largest private, not-for-profit medical center, a regional tertiary referral center, and nationally recognized for women's health and obstetrics, pulmonary care, and stroke treatment.

The same spirit of human kindness that brought Alta Bates to each patient's bedside at the close of each day inspires us still.

Underscoring these accomplishments is the Medical Center's strongest tradition: compassionate care. The same spirit of human kindness that brought Miss Bates to each patient's bedside at the close of each day inspires us still.

This volume documents the history of Alta Bates Summit Medical Center and the five hospitals from which it grew. But it is through the health of our patients and well-being of our community, the skilled hands of our staff and the hearts and minds of our legions of volunteers that the tale is best told. It is in each life we touch, now and for generations to come, that Alta Bates Summit's timeless traditions—and remarkable record of achievement—will prosper.

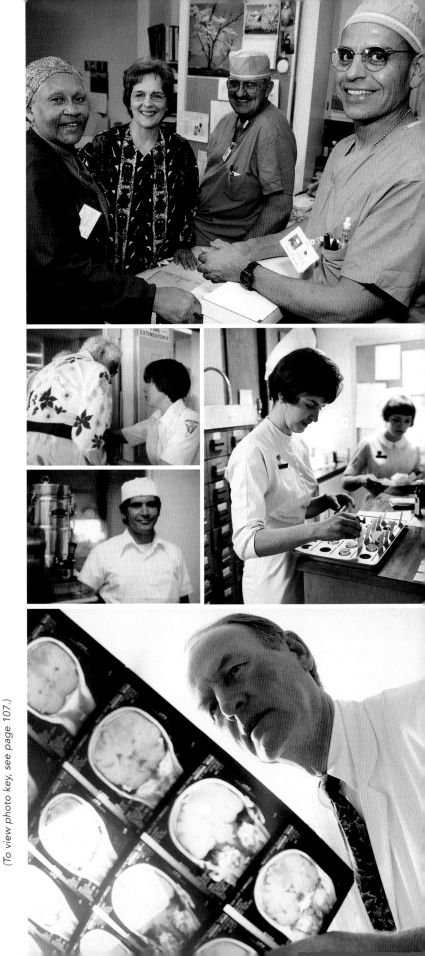

(To view photo key, see page 107.)

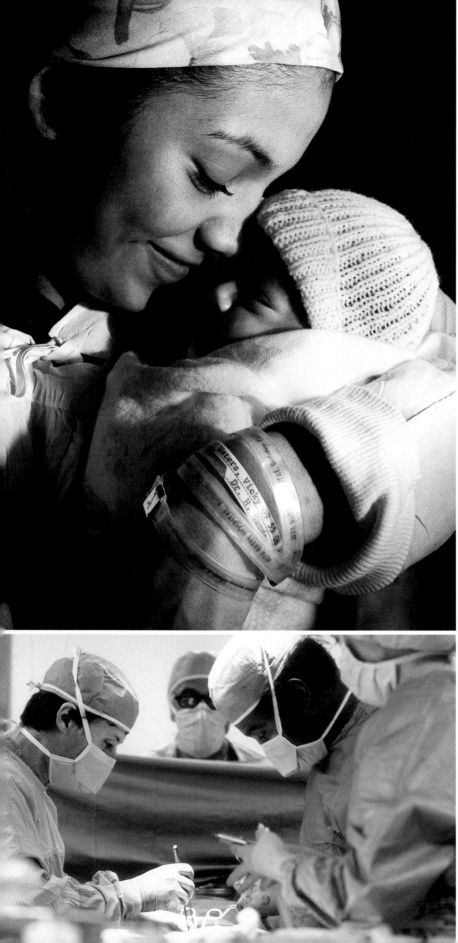
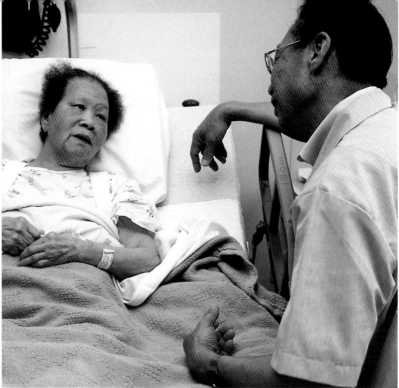
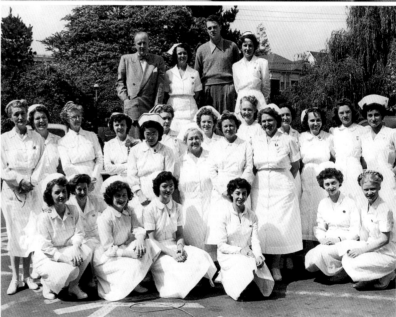
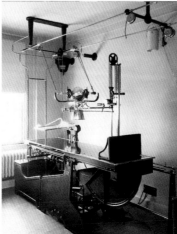
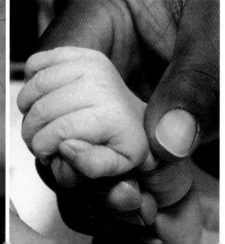

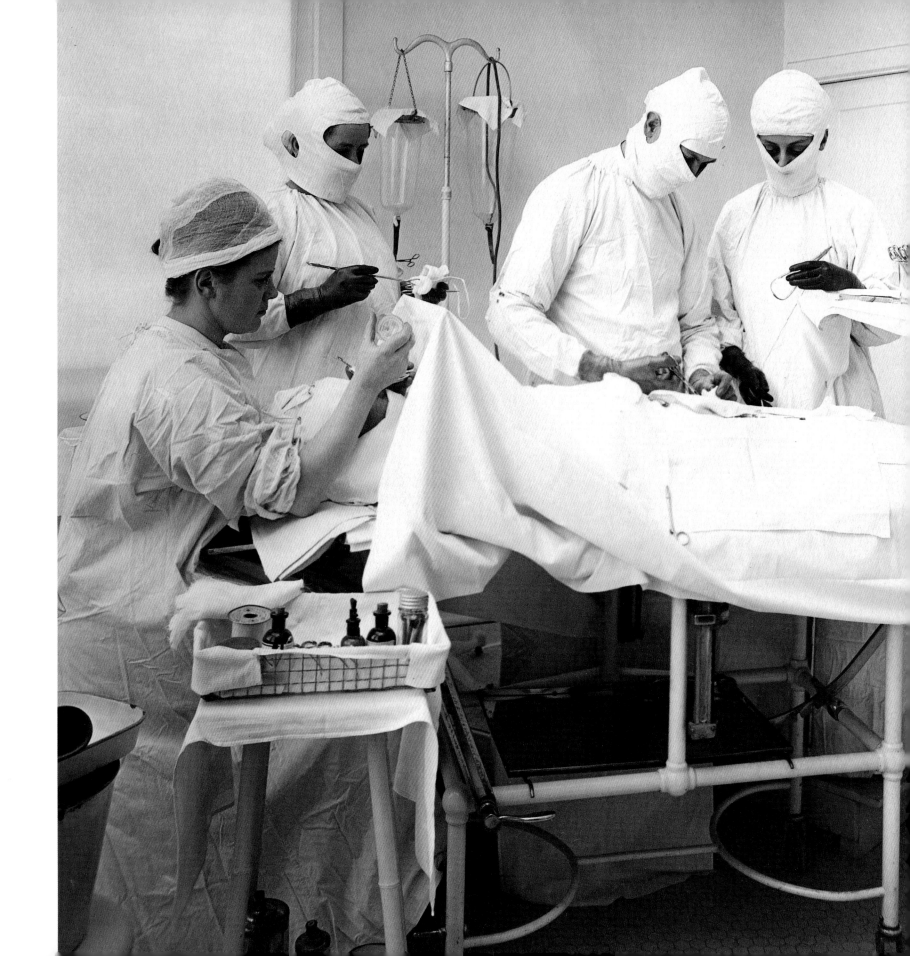

from these roots

Surgery at Alta Bates Hospital, 1920

At the turn of the 20th century, the cities of Oakland and Berkeley are coming of age. Yet their booming populations—inflated by former '49ers of the Gold Rush, heady pioneers fresh from the transcontinental railroad, and shaken refugees from San Francisco's Great Earthquake of 1906—outstrip their ability to mend the ill and afflicted. The need is great (and growing) for quality health care facilities and skilled medical professionals.

During the century's first decade, precursors of Alta Bates Summit Medical Center—Alta Bates, Roosevelt (later Berkeley General and then Herrick Memorial), Merritt, and Providence hospitals—open for patient care in the region. Peralta Hospital follows as the Roaring '20s come to a close.

In the intervening years, medical science witnesses tremendous progress. Physicians and patients begin to enjoy the benefits of earlier experimental breakthroughs, such as the X-ray in 1895 and blood typing in 1901. Rapid developments in medicine improve capabilities, including advances ranging from the introduction of the electrocardiograph to the discovery of insulin and penicillin.

Throughout their inaugural era, the community turns to these hospitals and trusts them in times of crisis. The hospitals rise to each occasion—tending to thousands of injured refugees from the Great Quake, treating hundreds stricken by the Spanish Influenza Epidemic, and relieving casualties from Berkeley's catastrophic 1923 fire. In their shining moments, the institutions establish their reputation and stand prepared for the many challenges ahead.

1890 Samuel Merritt, MD, wealthy real estate developer and influential entrepreneur-turned-politician, dies in Oakland at age 68. The former

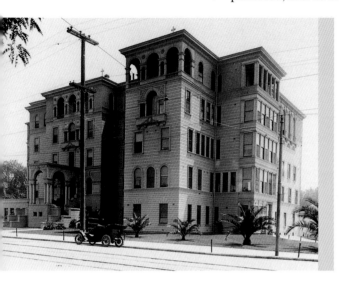

Providence Hospital

Mayor of Oakland leaves his $2 million estate to his widowed sister, Catherine Garcelon, with specific instructions to establish a trust to build "the most modern hospital facilities, staffed by competent personnel, to give the best possible care to both paying patients—those who can pay such reasonable costs as may be advised— and, by endowments to care for those worthy and valuable citizens ineligible for tax supported services, their care to be available free of all cost and expense, or on a part-pay basis."

1895 Physicist Wilhelm Roentgen discovers X-rays.

1900

1899 Aspirin (acetylsalicylic acid) is first marketed.

1901 Karl Landsteiner demonstrates blood typing, paving the way for the introduction of blood transfusions about six years later.

1902 The Providence Hospital Auxiliary is founded and supports early efforts to establish the hospital.

1903 The Wright brothers pioneer sustained, powered flights in a heavier-than-air machine.

1903 Alta Alice Miner Bates becomes the first graduate of the Eureka Training School for Nurses

in Eureka, California. Miss Bates eagerly pursues her calling when she moves with her family to Berkeley the next year and cares for a few patients in their 1318 Walnut Street home.

1904 **PROVIDENCE HOSPITAL OPENS.** After years of work by the Sisters of Providence, hundreds of Oakland citizens and prominent individuals, both clergy and lay, come to the completed hospital for the formal debut on April 5.

Hours before the 3 p.m. ceremony, the hospital's doors open to the public. They crowd its new corridors to inspect operating rooms, wards, and private rooms, all of which are furnished with the most modern equipment.

Assisted by the choir of sisters and a parish quartet, Archbishop Patrick Riordan begins the ceremonies by delivering the invocation and blessing the ground. San Francisco's Bishop George Montgomery, Oakland's Mayor Warren Olney, Judge Henry A. Melvin, City Attorney J.E. McElroy and Dr. Frank L. Adams follow with short addresses of gratitude and praise as they project the hospital's future impact on the city. Early the next morning, the Sisters of Providence open the hospital to the people of

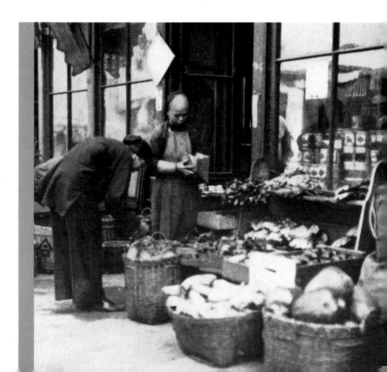

Oakland's Chinatown, 1911

founding visionaries

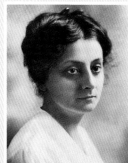

The proud history of Alta Bates Summit Medical Center begins with the inspiring tales of its founders. Here's how these extraordinary visionaries shaped their dreams for improving local health care:

SAMUEL MERRITT, MD Merritt purchased a 140-ton brigantine ship in his native New England, sailed around

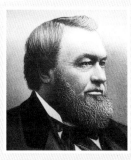

Valparaiso, Chile, and arrived in San Francisco the day after that city's great fire of 1850. He became a wealthy shipping and real estate magnate—spearheading construction of 125 buildings and Lake Merritt, organizing the Oakland Free Library, and serving as Mayor of Oakland and a University of California regent. He died in 1890, leaving a $2 million bequest to establish "the most modern hospital facilities" for the area's "worthy and valuable citizens," rich and poor alike. Construction of Samuel Merritt Hospital begins in 1905 (suffering damage in the '06 earthquake) and opens for patient care in 1909.

SISTERS OF PROVIDENCE In the early 1900s, two Sisters of Providence—Mother Mary Theresa and Sister Irene—arrive in Oakland to build a hospital at the request of the Archbishop of San Francisco and an Oakland Catholic priest. The leaders worry that Oakland's growing

population is taxing the community's ability to care for its sick and injured. They appeal to the Montreal-based Sisters of Providence, because the order had developed hospitals, schools, and orphanages in the Northwest. By January 1902, the Sisters have raised $12,000 to buy land at 26th Street and Broadway. When their hospital opens in April 1904, a dozen sisters join their Mother Superior in providing care.

LEROY FRANCIS HERRICK, MD The death of Herrick's wife motivated him to become an orderly and attend lectures at

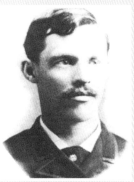

Lane Medical School (now Stanford). He later graduated from the University of Louisville medical school, mined gold in South Africa, and then opened a private medical practice in Oakland. Realizing Berkeley has no hospital, Dr. Herrick purchases a Victorian house at Dwight and Milvia streets and converts it into the 20-bed Roosevelt Hospital in 1904. The hospital is renamed Berkeley General Hospital in 1924 and later Herrick Memorial Hospital in 1945.

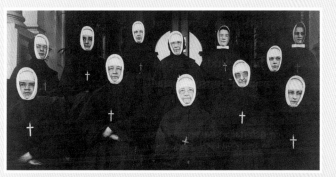

ALTA ALICE MINER BATES, RN Soft-spoken but determined, Miss Bates opens her parents' home to a few patients in 1904. Here, she hones her skills as a graduate of the Eureka Training School for Nurses. Area physicians are so impressed with her patient care, they urge the 25-year-old nurse to build a hospital. With $114 in cash, her father's architectural design, and credit from local merchants, Miss Bates founds the eight-bed Alta Bates Sanatorium at 2314 Dwight Way. Over the years she will serve as chief anesthetist, hospital administrator, and head of the nursing school, retiring in 1945.

THE "PERALTA FIVE" In the early 1920s, five prominent physicians—Drs. John L. Lohse, W.B. Palamountain, P.N. Jacobson, Hayward G. Thomas, and Quinton O. Gilbert—plan a private, physician-owned Oakland hospital and begin a

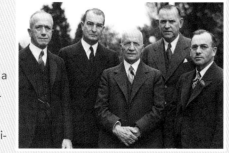

subscription drive. They explore constructing a new type of hospital that will combine stylish décor and architecture with modern medical equipment. Before the 120-bed facility opens in 1928, the name is changed from Hillcrest Hospital to Peralta Hospital in honor of Don Luis Maria Peralta on whose rancho many East Bay cities, including Oakland, now sit.

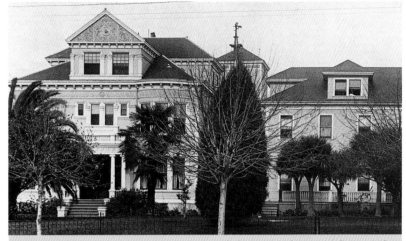

Roosevelt (later Herrick Memorial) Hospital

1905 The first Berkeley Public Library is built, with funds donated by the Andrew Carnegie Foundation.

1905 Vicks VapoRub is invented and novocaine is discovered. The year also witnesses the first artificial joint (hip). In 1905, Robert Koch, the founder of bacteriology, is honored for his discoveries of the tuberculosis and cholera bacteria.

1905 ALTA BATES SANATORIUM OPENS. To meet the growing medical needs of the Berkeley community—with the help of local businessmen and a good deal of credit—Miss Bates opens her eight-bed Alta Bates Sanatorium at 2314 Dwight Way and establishes a nursing school. "Here, she took 'four green women in white' and taught them dexterity in hand, mind and spirit to qualify them for nursing careers," the *Berkeley Gazette* would later write.

In the early days, there are as many as 10 physicians on staff. Miss Bates is chief anesthetist, hospital administrator, and head of the nursing school she founded. "Berkeley was never a town

Oakland following the same intentions of their founder, Mother Joseph: to maintain quality of life for anyone in need.

Over the course of those first 14 months, the sisters treat just over 1,000 patients, feed 400 needy in their dining room, and take food and money to numerous poor in their homes.

1904 ROOSEVELT HOSPITAL DEBUTS.
LeRoy Francis Herrick, MD, purchases one of Berkeley's larger mansions, the Hume House, and converts it into a 20-bed hospital. He names the facility Roosevelt Hospital, after Theodore Roosevelt for whom he had great admiration.

As with other hospitals of the time, boarding is as awkward as medical knowledge is vague. Patients are gingerly transported on stretchers up three flights of steps to the third floor for surgery. Facilities are strained and only 25 patients can be accommodated.

The hospital's early expansion is marked by the move of an old carriage house from the back of the grounds to a convenient location next to the original house. A small addition is also erected.

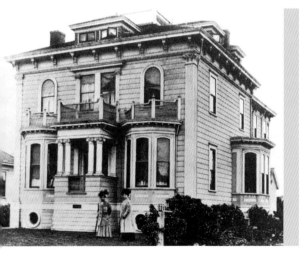

Alta Bates Sanatorium, 2314 Dwight Way, Berkeley, and its namesake and founder (left)

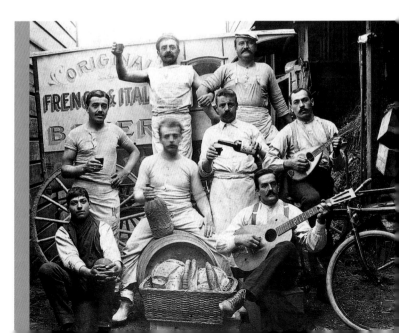

French-Italian bakery in West Oakland, circa 1900

content with less than the best. It was recognized from the start that the same graciousness that characterized Berkeley homes must also characterize Alta Bates Sanitorium [sic]," Raymond Young, president of Alta Bates' Board of Trustees will later observe in a 1956 hospital publication.

1906 The federal Food and Drug Administration is established.

1906 BAY AREA QUAKES. On April 18, San Francisco suffers a catastrophic earthquake and fire. Thousands of San Franciscans, including most of the injured, seek refuge in Oakland, which experiences scattered damage but remains standing. Many people and businesses permanently relocate in the East Bay and the region's population booms.

Over the next year, Oakland's population doubles, growing from 67,000 to 142,000. By 1909, the city's area almost triples from 22.9 to 60.25 square miles, as the residential districts of Claremont, Melrose, Fitchberg, and Elmhurst are incorporated. Berkeley's populace increases from 13,214 in 1900 to 40,434 in 1910—making it the nation's fourth fastest growing city.

1906 When the major ground shaking subsides, East Bay hospitals tend to the scores of injured who have crossed the San Francisco Bay to safety. At Providence, for example, the Sisters treat hundreds of casualties of the earthquake and feed thousands more.

A few miles away, tiny Alta Bates Sanatorium overflows with quake-stricken refugees. This same year, Miss Bates graduates her first class of six nurses.

1906–1907 Miss Bates and doctors in the community determine that her sanatorium isn't large enough to meet community needs, including those of quake-shy San Franciscans who have

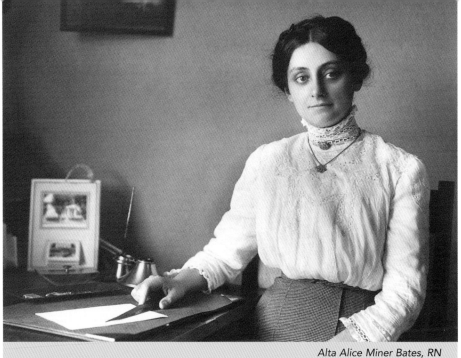

Alta Alice Miner Bates, RN

moved across the Bay. So she seeks a new site for a larger facility.

While exploring Berkeley one afternoon, she and her father find an ideal spot overlooking the Golden Gate. Stopping to talk with a man who is stacking lumber, they discover that he owns the property. It doesn't take long for Miss Bates to sell him her idea, and the following year she opens a new hospital at 2460 Webster Street. It has 12 beds, major and minor operating rooms, a delivery room, and quarters for her nursing students.

Lester Hink, one of Berkeley's top business executives, a philanthropist and later a hospital trustee, bestows generous gifts from his emporium to Miss Bates' new facility, including bed

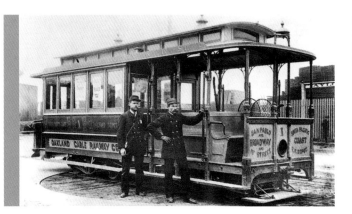

Cable cars in Oakland— not as famous as San Francisco's, but equally stylish

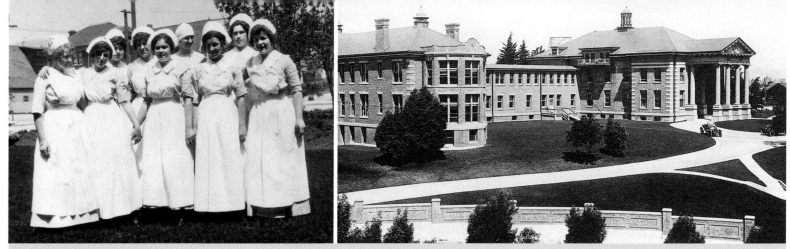

Alta Bates nursing students, circa 1914

Samuel Merritt Hospital

linens and blankets. "We were only too glad to extend credit to such a person," Hink would remark later.

Miss Bates moves next door to her hospital so that she can be only minutes away in case of emergencies. She serves as the hospital's anesthetist as well as teacher, nurse, and guiding force. One recollection about Miss Bates concerned her marvelous way with children who were undergoing surgery. She would recite Thorton Burgess' tale about Mother West Wind and have the children "blow and blow" along with her. They would go to sleep "blowing"; when they awoke they would ask to hear the rest of the story.

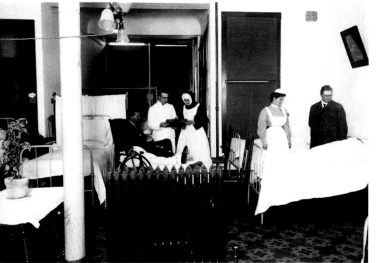

A Providence ward, 1905

1907 Providence School of Nursing graduates its first class.

1907 The Berkeley Chamber of Commerce begins its (unsuccessful) campaign to move the state capital to Berkeley.

The city of Berkeley is booming in the early 1900s, with businesses opening at a feverish pace, San Franciscans fleeing the ravages of the earthquake, and students arriving at record rates at the University. Of great significance is the extension of the Key System Transit Lines to the foot of University Avenue. It reduces commute time to San Francisco to a mere 36 minutes. Berkeley is now a viable commuter suburb of San Francisco and Oakland.

The new University of California sees its enrollment triple in the early 1900s, and international landmarks like the Campanile and Boalt Hall School of Law are built.

1907 A women's suffrage parade—the state's first —marches triumphantly through downtown Oakland. Women in California will win the right to vote in 1911.

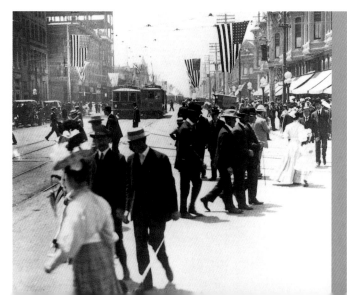

The vicinity of Broadway and 14th Street, Oakland

movers and shakers

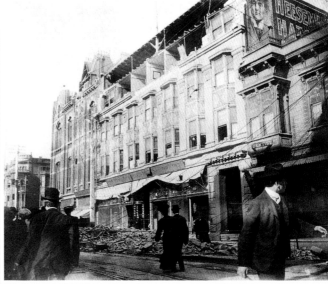

Oakland is spared major damage in the '06 quake.

San Francisco claims the fame in the Bay Area during the early 1900s. Contra Costa, as the East Bay was once known—including Oakland, a small city of 67,000, and Berkeley, a sleepy little college town—is an afterthought. That all changes one fateful spring morning in 1906.

At 5:13 a.m. on April 18, a massive earthquake shakes San Francisco. The temblor and ensuing three-day fire destroy much of the city and leave 225,000–250,000 homeless. Oakland and Berkeley are spared the brunt of the shocks but suffer damage. Oakland's 12th Street, just 14 blocks from Providence Hospital, sinks 18 inches; scores of homes slip off their foundations and storefronts collapse.

As San Francisco burns, more than 150,000 refugees crowd onto boats and escape to the East Bay. There, private businesses, individuals, hospitals, public agencies, and religious organizations rush to their aid. Makeshift relief camps are quickly established at Idora Park (a North Oakland amusement park) and nearby on Lake Merritt's shores. The Oakland Chinese community organizes a shelter for the 20,000 Chinese who flee San Francisco.

At Providence, the resourceful sisters move their 80 patients into sheltered, relatively undamaged areas and set up emergency beds and cots. Within days, they feed more than 2,000 people, shelter and treat hundreds of refugees, and distribute medicine to thousands.

The injured are also removed to medical facilities in Berkeley—Herrick Hospital (then Roosevelt Hospital) and Alta Bates Sanatorium, established in 1904 and 1905, respectively. A *Berkeley Gazette* columnist will later recall Miss Bates' heroics: "In the 2300 block on Dwight Way was a little sanitarium [sic]. Its patients were evacuated that drizzling April 18th morning when the building shook like a leaf but stood intact, except for the chimney. … During that week Miss Alta Bates was perhaps the busiest woman in Berkeley. And from that day on she has been a local institution herself."

After the quake, most refugees remain and many San Franciscans migrate, deciding it is safer on the other side of the Bay. As East Bay populations boom, so does demand for medical care. In response, Miss Bates builds a new 12-bed hospital in 1907, adding wings in 1910 and 1912. (Ironically, the earthquake also led to renovation of Oakland's Merritt Hospital. The temblor struck as Merritt was nearing completion, severely damaging its partially built south ward. When blueprints were lost in the San Francisco fire, architect Nathaniel Blaisdell was forced to redesign the structure and build it to meet post-earthquake codes requiring steel frames within brick walls.)

Only in hindsight will experts estimate that the historic temblor had registered 8.3 on the Richter scale. With the benefit of time, we can also now see that it was not the quake, but its cultural aftershock—the migration of hundreds of thousands of San Francisco's residents—that had the greatest impact on East Bay communities—and their hospitals.

Oakland Tribune *front page, April 18, 1906*

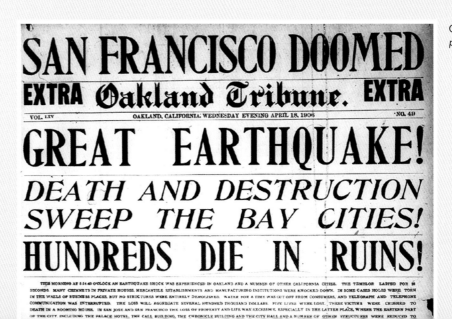

SAN FRANCISCO DOOMED
EXTRA Oakland Tribune. EXTRA
VOL. LXV   OAKLAND, CALIFORNIA. WEDNESDAY EVENING APRIL 18, 1906.   NO. 49

GREAT EARTHQUAKE!
DEATH AND DESTRUCTION SWEEP THE BAY CITIES!
HUNDREDS DIE IN RUINS!

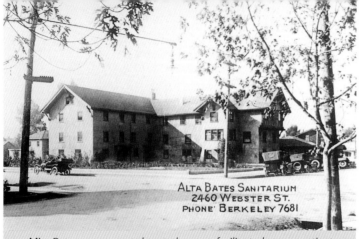

ALTA BATES SANITARIUM
2460 WEBSTER ST.
PHONE BERKELEY 7681

Miss Bates moves next door to her new facility to be near patients.

care to proper applicants who have their own physicians. Of the 549 patients admitted in 1909, 153 bills are paid by service endowment funds.

Merritt's school of nursing opens the same year, with dormitories occupying the south ward's second and third floors.

1908 Edna B. Shuey founds the Berkeley Health Center for the poor at 934 University Avenue.

1909 Vivian Rodgers becomes the first black to graduate from the University of California; August Vollmer is appointed Berkeley's first chief of police. The department will be the first ever to use the lie detector test in 1924.

1909 SAMUEL MERRITT HOSPITAL OPENS. The new Merritt opens for patient care, nearly three years after the '06 earthquake severely damaged its initial, nearly completed structure. The *Oakland Tribune* reports construction costs at $200,000.

Two of the first medical procedures in the new hospital: Drs. C.A. Dukes and M.L. Emerson upstage a planned first operation by a University of California physician in performing an "emergency" hemorrhoid surgery. Dr. Emerson delivers Merritt's first baby, Lois Merritt Peterson. The hospital empowers its superintendent to give free medical

1910 Oakland's population grows to 150,000—an increase of 83,000 in only four years.

1910 After the Mexican Revolution breaks out, nearly 10 percent of Mexico's population flee their homes to relocate in the American Southwest and California. They follow an earlier wave of Mexican laborers that began in 1869, working in Oakland's railroad freight yards, canneries, and garment factories.

1910 Alta Bates Hospital's new wing adds 24 beds. Quality care, always the hallmark of the medical facility, requires the addition of another new wing in 1912, increasing capacity to 36 beds. By now the nursing school is growing, and Miss Bates is becoming renowned for providing a homelike atmosphere in which patients know they are important.

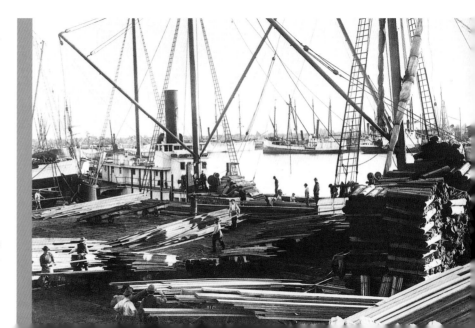

Oakland's harbor is its lifeblood, 1913.

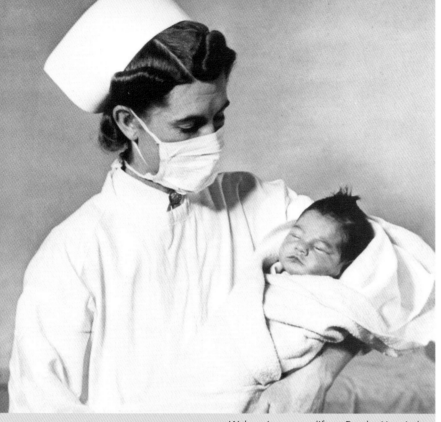

Welcoming a new life at Peralta Hospital

then second floor, administration building] were fixed at $4, $5 and $6, respectively."

October 4, 1910: "The S. was instructed to accept Obstetrical cases, using the four front rooms of the Administration Building, the rate being $50 per week for the same, or $7 a day; for 2 in a room, $4 a day. For Mother in room without the babe in the room, $6 a day."

April 25, 1911: "By unanimous vote it was agreed that no free case should be allowed to remain in the hospital more than five weeks without permission granted by the Trustees upon application of the attending physician through the Chief of Staff of that department."

Alta Bates not only signed this delivery room bill but also served as the anesthetist at the birth. The beneficiary of her services, little Philip Ferrier, will grow up to become a general surgeon at Alta Bates Hospital.

1910–1911 Excerpts from summaries of several administrative meetings at Merritt:

May 31, 1910: "Superintendent was instructed to learn just what arrangements the several 'ex-ray' [sic] experts of San Francisco had with their different hospitals, so as to form some idea of running when our ex-ray machine was set up."

May 31, 1910: "Superintendent was instructed to engage a good chef at $90 per month; chef to live in hospital if possible."

June 28, 1910: "Superintendent was requested to have monthly examinations of the milk made by our pathologist. S. was requested to order certified milk for the hospital."

August 25, 1910: "It was agreed that the charges (for X-ray) should be as follows: For making an X-ray plate and developing the same, $10; for an examination without a plate, $5."

Sept. 27, 1910: "The prices for rooms in the newly finished part of the hospital [the

1911 Mrs. Henrietta Farrelly gives the Merritt trustees $50,000 for construction of the Farrelly Home for Nurses, allowing nursing students to move out of the south ward and into their own dormitory—increasing the hospital's bed capacity to 75.

1911 The cost of a major operation at Merritt is $20.

1911 First laparoscopy (minimally invasive abdominal surgery) is performed at Johns Hopkins.

1911 Ishi, a Yahi man who was found in Oroville, comes to Berkeley where he will live for the remainder of his life, under the care of UC Berkeley anthropologist Alfred Kroeber.

(Bill for Philip's birth)

BILLS PAYABLE WEEKLY IN ADVANCE

Berkeley, Cal., Mar. 19-17

Mrs. W. W. Ferrier

To The Alta Bates Sanatorium Dr.

To wk ending Mar 26	$28 00
" Delivery room	5 00
	33 00

RECEIVED PAYMENT

Alta Bates

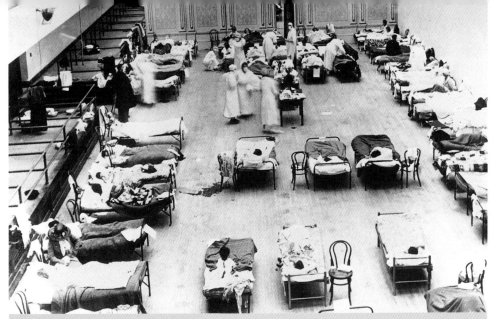

Hospitals stretch resources to care for victims of the 1918–1919 Spanish Flu Epidemic. Even the Oakland Auditorium is set up for emergency care.

American Cancer Society is founded—in a time when nine out of 10 people die of the disease.

1913 California passes the Alien Land Act, barring alien immigrants, primarily Japanese and other Asian/Pacific farmers, from leasing or owning land. States across the nation approve similar laws.

1914 "The Nurse," a poetic play on words published in *The Ward Carriage*, from Alta Bates School of Nursing:
Temperament always mild and serene,
Honesty of purpose forever is keen,
Earnestness marks each duty she performs.
Neatness is one of her personal charms,
Usefulness her one highest aim,
Right the motto she'll always maintain,
Smiles ever giving all night and all day,
Eternally with us, dear nurse, come and stay.

1914 Oakland's new City Hall debuts. The Beaux Arts–style structure is said to be the tallest building west of the Mississippi River and the first government building designed as a "skyscraper."

1911 Casimir Funk coins the term "vitamine" (later, vitamin) and is credited with the nutrient's discovery.

1912 School of Nursing at Samuel Merritt graduates its first class.

1912 Baby Hospital, later known as Children's Hospital, opens in Oakland.

1912 The luxury ocean liner Titanic sinks off the coast of Newfoundland. This same year, toys reportedly make their debut in Cracker Jacks boxes.

Operating room, Alta Bates, circa 1920s

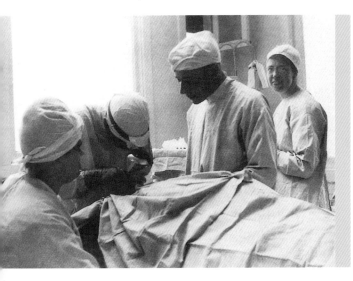

1913 The first Model T. Ford rolls off the assembly line. With a $550 price tag ($300 less than its less efficiently produced predecessor), it will become the first widely affordable, mass-produced car.

1913 First mammogram, by Dr. A. Salomon, is performed in Germany. The

1915 San Francisco celebrates the opening of the Panama Canal with the Panama Pacific International Exposition, attracting thousands of new residents to the East Bay.

1915 Miss Bates judges the area to be in need of larger, more modern medical facilities. She forms a corporation to raise funds and takes on partners (suppliers, doctors, nurses, and businesspeople headed by Lester Hink and Clarence Bullwinkel) to build a new hospital. Several hundred people buy

LAKESIDE PARK OAKLAND

A Sunday afternoon at Lake Merritt, 1910

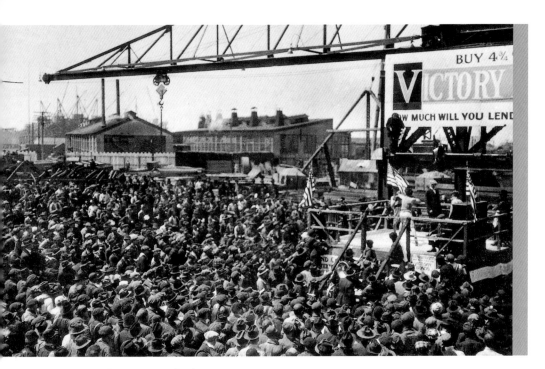

Rallying support back home for the troops in World War I

bonds or stock to support the effort. Many prominent physicians join the staff.

1915 Alameda County Infirmary, founded in 1864, becomes Fairmont Hospital.

1915–1925 Dutch physiologist Willem Einthoven refines the first electrocardiogram into a form used for decades.

1917 WORLD WAR I HITS HOME. The United States declares war on Germany and enters World War I.

1917 When the United States enters the war in Europe, Miss Bates trains Red Cross volunteers as well as student nurses. The nursing school now has 22 pupils— their hours are long and their pay is $5 a day. She is strict, but that's why students come to Alta Bates to train.

1917 Frederick M. Loomis, MD, brings anesthesiology equipment to Oakland's

Fabiola Hospital (founded in 1876) for use in an obstetrical case. This is the first such use in the West. Later, Dr. Loomis becomes a Peralta Hospital staff physician and well-known author.

1918–1919 Spanish Influenza Epidemic strikes the nation. An estimated 500,000–675,000 die in the United States, 25 million worldwide.

1918–1919 INFLUENZA EPIDEMIC RAGES. During the flu epidemic, thousands contract the disease, which spreads unhampered for many months. All available Oakland medical and nursing personnel work around the clock, either at their own facilities or at the new Oakland Auditorium, which has been turned into a makeshift emergency care facility.

Providence fills its 100 beds and also cares for the many ailing patients who crowd into hallways and parlors.

Ella Hagar, a civic leader, Alta Bates advisory trustee, and daughter of University of California at Berkeley president David P. Barrows, will recall how everyone wore face masks to avoid the flu during the epidemic: "I remember that the dean of women wore a pink silk one."

The flu left its impact on Alta Bates as well. The February 1954 issue of *R.N.* will later report: "Patients were arriving and dying so fast that there was scarcely time to prepare a room for the next patient. Two-thirds of the nursing and medical staff were in bed with flu or pneumonia, the laundry workers were few and far between, and Ling, the cook, was barely able to keep going. But [Miss] Bates walked calmly onto the third floor with a yellow mixing bowl from her own kitchen."

According to the article, Miss Bates mixed mustard paste while the few remaining nurses spread it on gauze and wrapped it with a hot water bottle to keep it warm until it could be

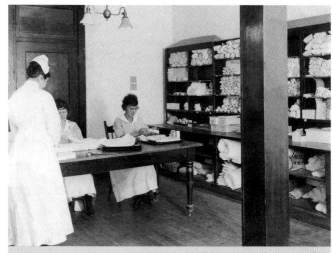

A 1920 supply room, predecessor of modern central processing

placed on the patient's chest—the only treatment for the flu in 1918.

1919 Excerpts from a May 6 inspection report, Alta Bates:

Bed capacity: 40

Total number of patients in Medical, Surgical and Obstetrical services during 1918: 1200

Obstetrical Services: 383

Medical Service: 116

Monthly average operations: 95

Daily average number of patients: 36

Children: very few (affiliation with Baby Hospital, Oakland, three months)

Contagious Services: none

Psychopathic Service: none

Tuberculosis: none

General appearance of Hospital is excellent. ...

Private Rooms: Private rooms are comfortably furnished; regulation hospital bed; good mattresses and bedding; floors clean; general appearance of rooms, very good. ...

Operating Room: The operating room was found very busy on the day of inspection. Condition of operating room, excellent; equipment, excellent. Three students on duty.

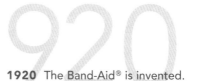

1920 The Band-Aid® is invented.

1920 Women win the right to vote in the United States.

1920–1925 Berkeley has become quite the college football town. Andy Smith and his Wonder Team not only go undefeated this season, but outscore opponents 510 to 14! The team goes on to win 50 games in a row, including five wins over rival Stanford.

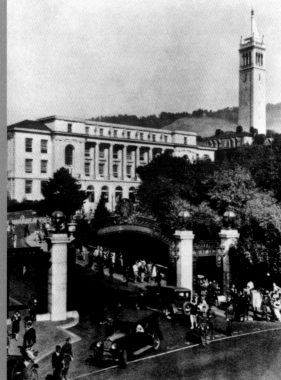

Above: The view from the University of California's Sather Gate, 1920
Below: Old City Hall stands in front of the new in this panoramic shot at Broadway and 14th Street.

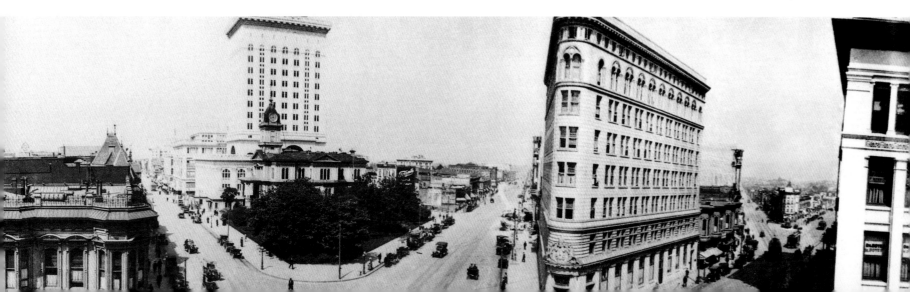

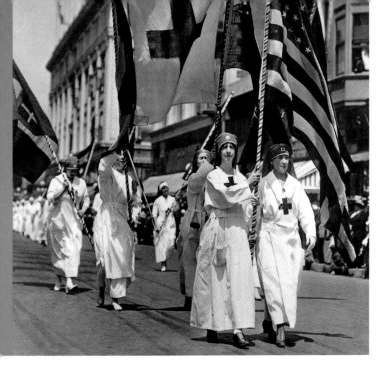

A jubilant
Red Cross parade

1920 Oakland's Sisters of Providence set their sights on constructing a new hospital. They spot a likely parcel of land (bounded by Central Avenue, Summit, and Webster, at what would become 30th Street) and offer to purchase it from the owner, Arthur Breed Sr. His stately, three-story Victorian home stands at the center of the property surrounded by enormous lawns and gardens.

Over the next six years, local banks and the Archdiocese loan a good portion of the amount needed. The still-fresh memories of Oakland's inadequate health care facilities, prompted by the Spanish Influenza Epidemic, spurs scores of private citizens and organizations to contribute unprecedented support. The Auxiliary sponsors card parties with admission fees donated to the new building fund; the student nurses hold raffles and raise the greatest part of the cost for the Pediatric Department; doctors donate money for specific equipment; the parish of St. Francis de Sales holds fundraising campaigns; and private citizens of varying means give large and small donations.

1921 Sir Frederick Banting and Charles Best discover insulin. Banting wins the 1923 Nobel Prize in Medicine.

1921 Oakland has become the greatest freight terminal west of Chicago. It is now the terminus of three transcontinental railroads, as well as many shipping lines.

The city experiences a dizzying growth rate in the '20s, accelerated by 7,000 newcomers each year.

— THEN AND NOW —

ambulances

Help is on the way: Berkeley's first Emergency Department is founded at the hospital later known as Herrick Memorial and proudly features ambulance service (left). With the benefit of vehicles sporting far greater horse power, Alta Bates Summit Medical Center's Emergency Departments will later become invaluable assets in the East Bay. More than 80,000 visits will be recorded in 2004.

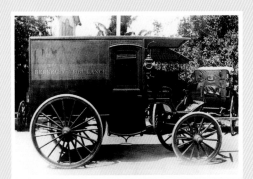

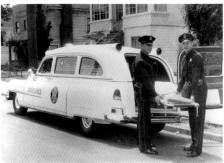

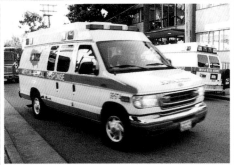

TEL {MERRITT 511. OAKLAND AMBULANCE CO.
     {B 1162   GRANT D. MILLER, PROP 1186 EAST 14TH ST.
                                         OAKLAND, CAL.

This growth is sustained by new manufacturing concerns that create a 40 percent increase in Oakland's gross product and employ 19,000 industrial workers. Real estate developers overtake the city and build scores of new housing tracts; construction permits in 1925 total $39 million.

1922 Maxwell Hallauer receives a license for Berkeley's first radio station. He opens a studio in the Claremont Hotel and uses the call letters KRE.

1923 The Berkeley Health Department creates a public health program, hiring 13 nurses—the first such program in the United States. In Oakland, the Visiting Nurses Association is formed.

1923 FIRESTORM DEVASTATES. On September 17, at about noon, smoke begins to billow over the top of the Berkeley Hills in what will become Tilden Park. Within a few minutes, burning leaves, grass, and shingles have whipped down the hills, and there isn't enough water to stop the flaming advance. Before it is over, 584 family residences, apartment houses, fraternity and sorority houses, and a fire house will be destroyed and 100 more buildings damaged. Alta Bates Hospital overflows with patients suffering burns and injuries. *The Berkeley Voice* will later estimate the disaster's price tag at $10 million.

1923 The Peralta Hospital Association begins when a group of Oakland physicians gather to discuss the East Bay hospital shortage. Other physicians will later join these doctors and prominent citizens to develop the planning and financing toward purchase of the Campbell Estate, the Peralta site.

1924 Roosevelt is renamed Berkeley General Hospital when a new two-story concrete wing is

building a tradition
1904–1928

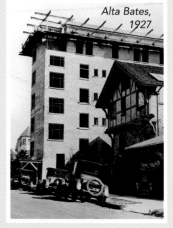

Alta Bates, 1927

ALTA BATES

1905 Eight-bed, 14-room sanatorium, 2314 Dwight Way
1907 Twelve-bed, three-story hospital and quarters for nursing students, 2460 Webster Street
1910 New wing, now 24-bed capacity
1912 New wing increases capacity to 36 beds.
1928 $750,000, six-story, 112-bed building at 3000 Regent Street

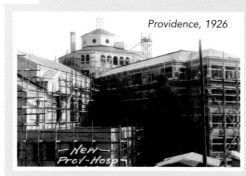

Providence, 1926

—New Prov-Hosp

HERRICK

1904 Hume House converts to Roosevelt Hospital at Dwight Way and Milvia Street
1924 Renamed Berkeley General; new two-story, concrete wing and 50-bed capacity

MERRITT

1905 The hospital and nursing school construction begins in the Academy Hill area.
1906 The earthquake severely damages nearly completed structure.
1909 The 36-bed hospital and nursing school open.
1927 First major expansion; boosts bed capacity to 119

PERALTA

1928 Construction of plush, 120-bed facility on Orchard Avenue (now 30th Street)

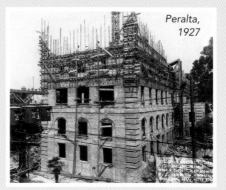

Peralta, 1927

Work crew, 1928

PROVIDENCE

1904 The Sisters move into the new building at 26th and Broadway.
1926 The new Providence is built on Orchard Avenue and Summit Street, seven times the original building's size.

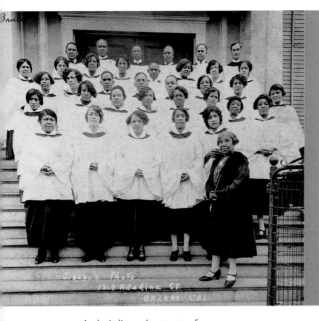

A choir lines the steps of First African Methodist Episcopal Church, 1920.

Left: The Oakland Police Department enforces Prohibition during the 1920s, under the leadership of District Attorney Earl Warren (who will later become Chief Justice of the U.S. Supreme Court). Right: The Berkeley Firestorm of 1923 destroys 584 buildings.

added onto the west side. The new 50-bed capacity grows to 100 beds by a decade later.

1924 The first disposable handkerchief is made in the United States. It's first called cellwipes and later dubbed Kleenex®.

1925 Albert Calmette vaccinates children against tuberculosis using BCB (nonvirulent bovine culture).

1925 C.L. Dellums helps set up the Brotherhood of Sleeping Car Porters, the nation's first African American trade union. Seventy years later, Oakland's picturesque train station is named in Dellums' honor.

1925

1925 Highland Hospital, an Alameda County facility, opens in Oakland.

1926 Crowds flock to the opening of Oakland's Grand Lake Theater and enjoy its Wurlitzer's wondrous melodies.

1926 THE NEW PROVIDENCE OPENS. The debut of the hospital and the new Providence College of Nursing is an auspicious occasion. In two hours, seven ambulances convey 75 patients to a building seven times the size of the original hospital and just a few blocks away.

Perched upon the little hill overlooking Oakland, and now remote from the noise of Broadway's bustling traffic, the bright, new hospital enjoys a great serenity. Ironically, a tremor jars the earth the following morning. "Our fine new building shook like a little flower," writes Sister Angelica in the *Chronicles,* the Sisters' official log of hospital happenings. Not a bit of damage occurs.

The construction plans called for a cruciform-style building. From a huge octagonal center column, which gives each floor a central rotunda, four wings spread in a cross-like fashion to each end corner of the lot. At the end of each wing, solariums on every floor overlook Oakland and the San Francisco Bay. To spare patients some hospital noise, the central rotundas serve as the main hubs of activity where nurses' stations, elevators, entrances, exits, and all service rooms are located.

The Sisters planned to double the capacity to 225 beds and have 75 more available; create large service areas for Pharmacy, Physiotherapy, X-ray, Cardiology, and Pathology Departments; and

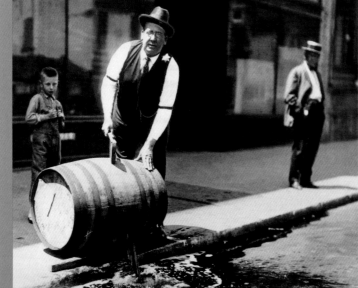

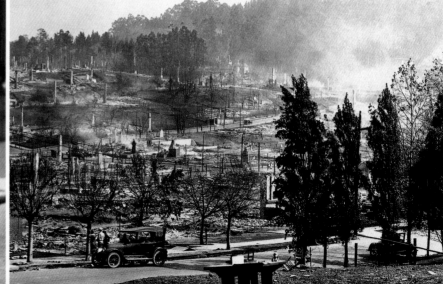

*Merritt clinical laboratory, circa 1926;
foreground, Robert Glenn, MD*

reserve a major portion of one wing for a Children's Department. A one-story, double stairway was built to elevate the main entrance, which was designed to overlook 30th Street. Accompanying these plans were ambitious designs for the adjacent student nurses' residence, a four-story school and dormitory.

After so many years of fire destruction in the city, the hospital's builders adhered strictly to the newest building ordinances for hospital construction, incorporating the latest techniques in fireproofing and placing fire escapes at the end of each wing. Under two wings they built basements comprised of various areas designed specifically for cold storage of food; sterilization of mattresses, clothing, and dressings; storage of supplies and records; and an autopsy room. On the fifth floor they built a glass-enclosed roof garden and an open-air veranda for convalescing patients.

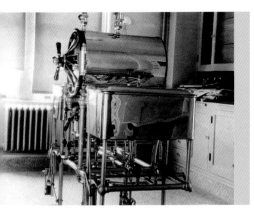

Sterilization equipment, Providence

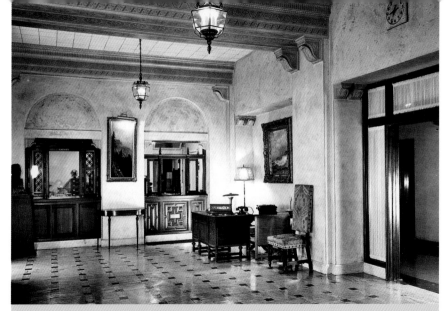

The opulent lobby at the newly constructed Peralta, 1928

1927 Merritt's most expensive room, with connecting bath, costs $10 a day, according to a 1974 *Merritt Monogram*. Adding a private bath costs $1 extra. Other vital statistics:
Ward rates: $5 a day
Children's Ward: $4 a day
Nursery's special "babe alone" rate: $2.50
Regular rates included "general nursing care, board, dressings and medicines of the United States Pharmacopeia and routine laboratory service."

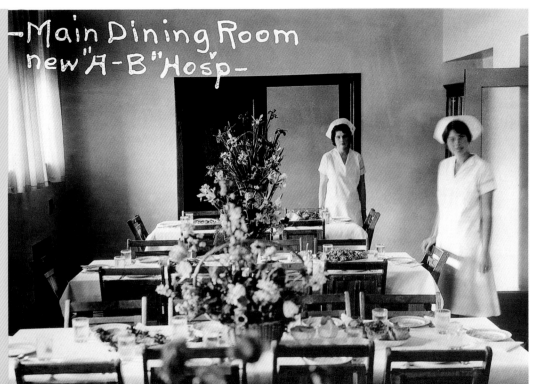

The finest in hospital dining at the new Alta Bates, circa late 1920s–early 1930s

—Main Dining Room new "A-B" Hosp—

1927 Aboard the Spirit of St. Louis, Charles Lindbergh makes the first solo trans-Atlantic flight. This same year, Lindbergh presides at the dedication of the Oakland Municipal Airport. An expanded airport, renamed Oakland International Airport, will open in 1962.

1927 Merritt undergoes its first major expansion, adding a two-story wing and boosting its capacity to 119 beds.

1928 The ability of hemoglobin to combine with oxygen (thus enabling it to transport airborne gas to tissue) is demonstrated by Joseph Barcroft in his *The Respiratory Function of Blood*.

1928 A NEW, EXPANDED ALTA BATES OPENS. The Roaring '20s leaves its mark on everything, including the elaborate opening festivities of Alta Bates' new $750,000 hospital. City authorities close the street for dedication ceremonies. Werner Hoyt, MD, and Dexter Richards Sr., MD, fly over the scene in a tiny biplane. While Dr. Hoyt pilots, Dr. Richards tosses masses of flower petals below onto Miss Bates and her gathered guests.

Medical care truly remains an important local priority—and Alta Bates' facilities, equipment, and number of beds continue to increase at an unprecedented rate. The new fireproof facility, designed by architect Clarence C. Cuff and financed by bonds sold to the community, boasts

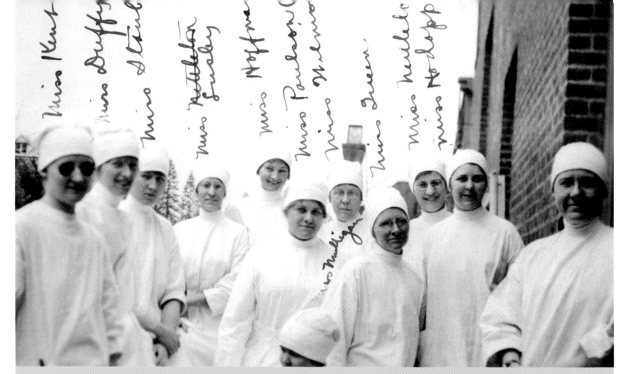

A personalized portrait of Providence nurses

the latest medical equipment and 112 beds. Its soundproof partitions, comprised of gypsum and rice hulls, are poured into patented steel forms. This is the first hospital on the West Coast to adopt this method, which was found to provide extra fire protection. By design, the operating room is located on the top floor so that plenty of fresh air and sunlight can stream into the room—considered a modern convenience at the time.

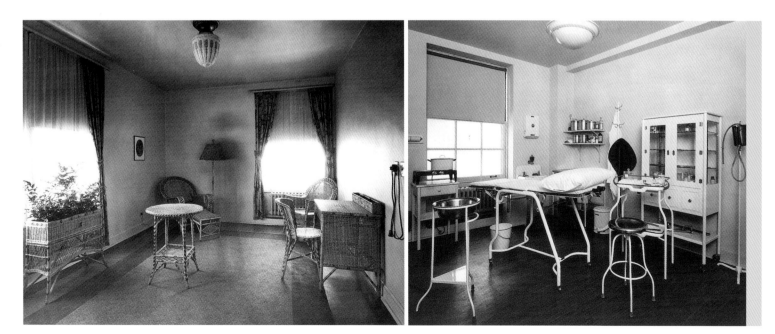
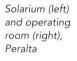

Solarium (left) and operating room (right), Peralta

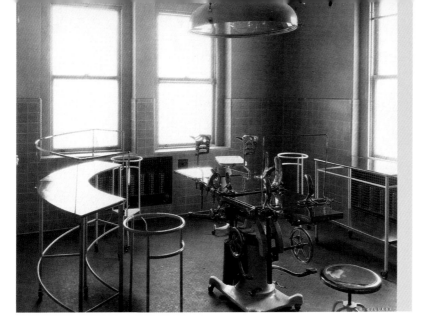

Access to fresh air as in this Alta Bates surgical suite (circa late 1920s–early 1930s) is considered good medical practice.

Females of all ages flock to Oakland's Grand Lake Theater for Ladies Matinee, circa 1920s

every conceivable aid to medical science in a building that has the appearance and atmosphere of a private residence."

Always concerned about her patients' comfort, Miss Bates has each room painted a different pastel shade with colored glass light fixtures to match, in recognition of the therapeutic value of color. The community reciprocates, with deepening respect and affection for Miss Bates. Some 75 years later, Francis Hanna, a retired nurse, volunteer, and trustee at Alta Bates, would vividly recall, "I came to this hospital in 1929. It was brand new, just a couple of years after it was built. People used to drive around on a Sunday just to see the hospital and walk through."

An early *Berkeley Daily Gazette* enthuses: "From the imposing entrance at 3000 Regent St. and the marquise covered ambulance entrance on Webster St. to the water storage tanks with water softening apparatus and sterilizers under the mission tiled roof, the six stories represent

1928 PERALTA OPENS. Peralta, named after the Spanish family who once owned much of the East Bay, opens its doors as a 120-bed, acute-care

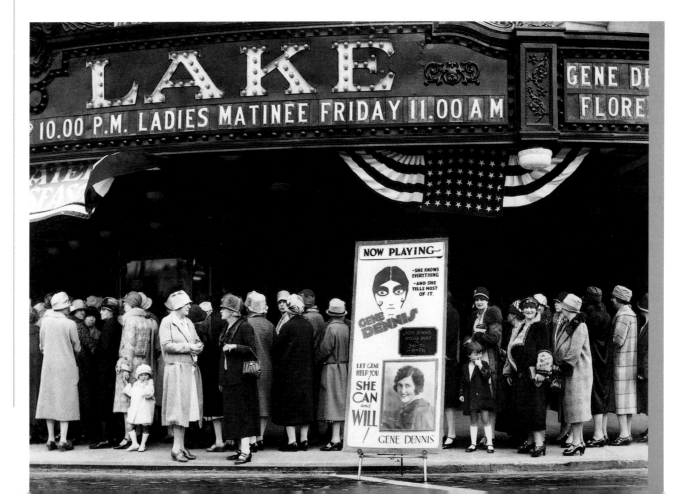

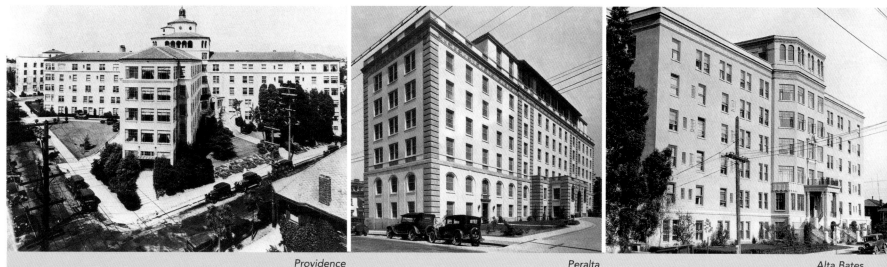

Providence   Peralta   Alta Bates

facility. Five Oakland physicians band together to create the distinctive medical institution that is erected on Orchard Street (now 30th), between Broadway and Telegraph.

The first Peralta patient is its architect, William Corlett. John L. Lohse, MD, co-founder, performs the first surgery. Albert Rowe Sr., MD, refers Peralta's first nonceremonial patient, who is in a diabetic coma. Treatment, which is successful, consists of a salt and sugar compound, mixed by pharmacist George Wood and administered intravenously. Wood—who will later become hospital administrator and, as a retiree, president of Peralta Medical Foundation—is paid $200 a month plus meals to run the pharmacy. This same day, Ruth Ann Woodson is the first baby born at Peralta.

1928 Alexander Fleming discovers penicillin.

1928 For the first time in the city's history, traffic signals are installed to control the congestion in Oakland's bustling downtown.

1929 The Stock Market crashes and the Great Depression begins.

1929 Percy William Leopold Camp uses epinephrine in the form of an inhaler for asthma. Carl Peter Henrik Dam (Denmark) discovers the antihemorrhagic factor (vitamin K) for which he will share the Nobel Prize in 1943.

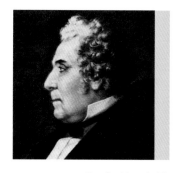

1929 PROVIDENCE'S PART-PAY CLINIC OPENS. The clinic, the first in the East Bay, is created for mothers who don't have the necessary funds for maternity and pediatric care. The clinic offers prenatal care, delivery, and one year of postnatal care, payable on a sliding scale, according to income. When it opens, the base rate for the entire package of services is $25, but during the Depression and World War II, Providence's clinic will care for thousands of mothers and infants, many of whom can pay nothing.

1929 To make way for new homes, razing begins of Idora Park, North Oakland's 17-acre, 25-year-old amusement park (in the vicinity of 57th and Shattuck).

Peralta Hospital is named in honor of Don Luis Maria Peralta, whose 1820 land grant included vast territory that would be occupied by Oakland, Berkeley, Emeryville, Piedmont, Alameda, Albany, and part of San Leandro. Pictured here: Don Jose Vicente Peralta, one of the heirs of the original Rancho San Antonio whose holdings included the future Pill Hill.

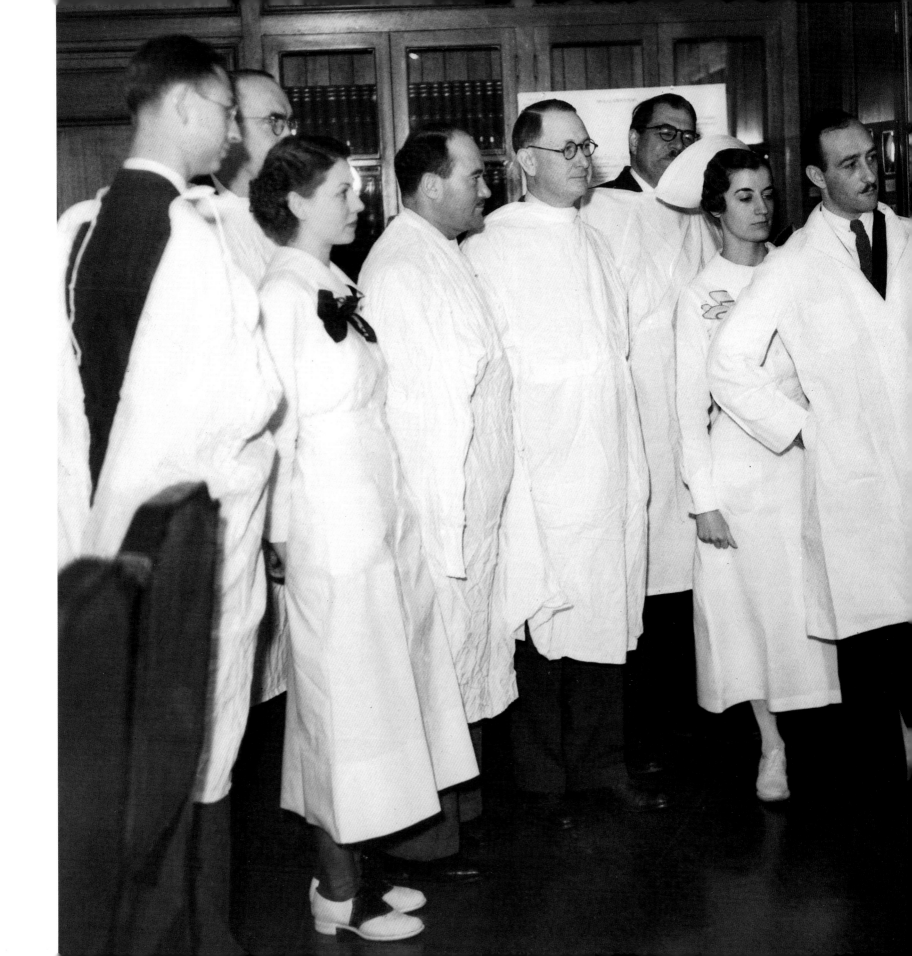

through crisis and war

Touring the facilities at Peralta Hospital

The 1930s and 1940s are a roller-coaster experience for Oakland and Berkeley, marked first by the economy's historic downturn, then by global conflagration, and finally—gratefully—by declarations of peace.

As ever, the fate of East Bay hospitals swings with the times. They, too, are jeopardized by the 1929 stock market crash and ensuing Great Depression that bankrupts millions of Americans and closes 45 percent of the nation's banks. Local medical institutions cut back services, practice cost-cutting measures, and find benefactors just to stay afloat.

World War II also puts a dramatic strain on area hospitals' resources. Hundreds of thousands of war workers pour into the region, while droves of doctors and nurses (in record numbers) answer their nation's call. Later, a 1948 California Department of Public Health report warns that hundreds will die due to lack of hospital facilities, and singles out Berkeley as having the fewest hospital beds per capita among major U.S. cities.

Despite the travails of this period, the field of medicine is uplifted by many breakthroughs. The world witnesses the first blood bank, kidney dialysis machine, MRI, pap smear test—even the first Alka Seltzer®. Locally, Berkeley becomes a focal point of scientific research. Ernest O. Lawrence, father of the cyclotron, wins the prestigious Nobel Prize for Physics in 1939, the first ever for a Cal professor. Alta Bates, Herrick, Merritt, Peralta, and Providence hospitals are revitalized by clinical discoveries and peacetime optimism, setting the stage for the era of unprecedented growth and prosperity that the '50s, '60s, and '70s will bring.

1930

1930s Alta Bates Hospital survives the financial crises sparked by the Great Depression, but still faces serious financial problems. Wages are cut 10 to 20 percent, but by 1938 Alta Bates (the hospital and the person) faces bankruptcy.

Once again, the community responds boldly and buys the hospital for $400,000. This dramatic action saves the medical facility and furthers the founder's vision for its future.

Over the years, Miss Bates' reputation will grow in the medical and lay community. She becomes known as the quintessential professional in appearance and demeanor—conscientiously making rounds each day and personally checking on each patient. As the story goes, the hospital founder once walked into a young woman's room and introduced herself saying, "Good evening, I'm Alta Bates," prompting the young lady to retort, "Oh yes? Well, I'm Sather Gate [the University of California landmark]."

"She had the respect of everyone," Elena Griffing, a 55-year Alta Bates employee, will observe in 2003. "When Miss Bates was here, she was so visible all the time. She was [always] walking the halls. I swear that lady never sat down. … Her uniform was starched so stiff she could stand it in a corner. She never had a wrinkle in it!"

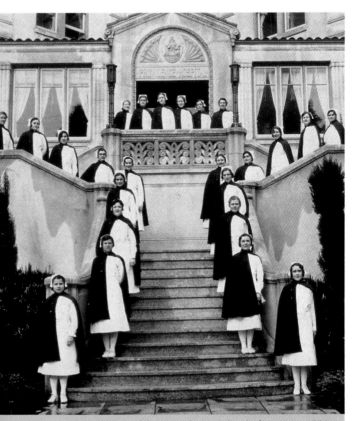

Proud graduates of the Providence School of Nursing, 1931

1930 OPERATING ROOM FEES—ALTA BATES

Minor	*$2.50 to $5*
Major	*$7.50 to $15*
Anaesthetic [sic]:	
Ether	*No charge*
Nitrous Oxide and Oxygen	*$6 per hour*

Anaesthetist [sic]: in discretion of anaesthetist. We do not employ technicians.

1930s Berkeley General Hospital (later renamed Herrick Memorial Hospital) is in rough financial straits when founder LeRoy Francis Herrick, MD, dies in 1932. Fortunately, his granddaughter's husband, Alfred Maffly, assumes control and, in 1935, convinces Dr. Herrick's heirs to donate the hospital's assets to a new, voluntary, not-for-profit, charitable organization, the Herrick Foundation. The estate at this time is valued at $500,000.

1930s To maximize help to the thousands of needy during the '30s economic downturn and yet manage the hospital's operating expenses, the Sisters of Providence seek new approaches to administration. Over the next few years, they will lease the hospital's X-ray department and pathology lab, reduce surgical and lab charges, and lower the ward bed rate. At the height of the Depression, 15,000 people are given free meals. The Sisters continue this practice during the pre-World War II years, feeding over 10,000 needy every year until 1940.

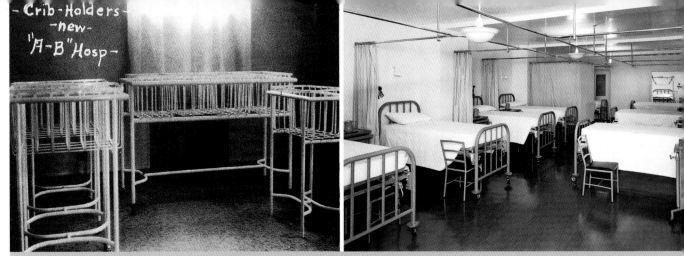

Baby gear, Alta Bates Hospital, circa late 1920s–early 1930s

The men's ward of Peralta, 1935

1930s Under President Robert Gordon Sproul, the University of California takes its place among the nation's educational giants. In this era, Professor Ernest O. Lawrence establishes his Radiation Laboratory at Cal. He and his colleagues in the emerging field of high-energy physics experiment with the first cyclotrons. (The original model of the cyclotron was said to be made of wire and sealing wax and probably cost $25 in all.)

Prior to this invention, the scope of nuclear medicine was severely limited by the scarcity of naturally occurring radioactive isotopes (special forms of atomic elements which emit radioactive rays). Lawrence's atom smasher, as it was then called, will make sufficient quantities of these substances available for medical purposes.

1930 More than 19 million people travel between the East Bay and San Francisco aboard ferries.

1931 Oakland's Paramount Theater opens—it's said to be one of the last of the Depression era's grand movie palaces.

1931 Financial crisis notwithstanding, new physicians gravitate to Berkeley. Among them is Hubert Long, MD, a beloved Berkeley pediatrician, whose many efforts on behalf of the hospital are acknowledged when Alta Bates' nursery is dedicated in his honor. "The goal of almost any young doctor coming to Berkeley was to have the distinction of becoming a member of the Alta Bates Medical Staff," Dr. Long will later observe. "It had the reputation of high standards and genuine care for patients."

1931 Alka Seltzer® is marketed as a remedy for headache and upset stomach.

1932 The first blood bank is established, in Leningrad, USSR. The first such facility in the United States starts up in Chicago in 1937.

1932 Fabiola Hospital, originally known as Oakland Homeopathic Hospital and Dispensary and the city's first general hospital, is closed at its Broadway and Moss Avenue (now MacArthur Boulevard) location. Fabiola's founding had been spearheaded 56 years earlier by 18 women who

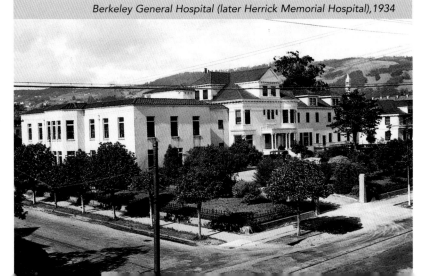

Berkeley General Hospital (later Herrick Memorial Hospital), 1934

"each gave $50 and an unlimited amount of energy and enthusiasm to the establishment of a hospital for the worthy, nonindigent poor and for those of limited means and no home," according to Milton Henry Shutes, MD, in his 1946 *History of the Alameda County Medical Association.*

Fabiola's new maternity building and real estate is given to Samuel Merritt Hospital, because Merritt comes nearest to paralleling its own benevolent program. Merritt trustees ultimately sell the Fabiola building and property in 1942, applying the proceeds toward construction of the North Wing in 1952.

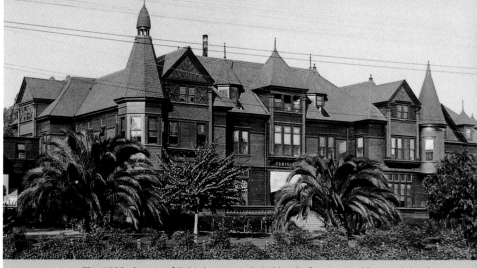

The 1932 closure of Fabiola Hospital, Oakland's first general hospital, leads to transfer of its maternity building and land to Merritt Hospital.

Some things never change: Traffic clogs Berkeley's bustling Telegraph Avenue.

1933 THE GREAT DEPRESSION DEEPENS.
At the nation's economic ebb, more than 11,000 of its 24,000 banks have failed, destroying depositors' savings. Millions of people are out of work and seeking jobs. (In the '30s, unemployment hits 25–30 percent.) Additional millions work at subsistence-level jobs. Currency values drop and farm markets erode.

1933 Ascorbic acid (vitamin C) is synthesized by Polish chemist Tadeus Reichstein.

1933 Construction begins on the Golden Gate Bridge and the San Francisco-Oakland Bay Bridge. When the Bay Bridge opens to traffic on November 12, 1936, ceremonies last four days; the bridge toll starts at 65 cents and is lowered to 25 cents by 1940. The Golden Gate Bridge will open May 27, 1937.

1933 The Isom triplets are born at Merritt. This same year, Merritt's medical staff places a special bronze plaque on the crypt of hospital founder Samuel Merritt, MD, in Mountain View Cemetery. (Merritt was one of the cemetery's organizers and its first president.)

1933 Peralta's Board of Trustees appoints George U. Wood, hospital pharmacist, as acting administrator of the then financially troubled hospital. On Wood's recommendation, Peralta reorganizes in the mid-'30s as a not-for-profit corporation with a voluntary board of directors. Thanks to Wood's successful belt-tightening measures, bank loans are paid off and bonds retired within seven years.

1934 *Peralta Hospital Rates, from the 1934 Bulletin of Peralta Hospital:*

Medical and Surgical (per day)	
Four-bed room	*$4.50, $5*
Two-bed room	*$5, $6*
Private room	*$6, $7.50, $9*
Industrial Cases (four-bed room)	*$3.50*
Children's Ward	*$4*
Obstetrical Service private room	*$8.50, $9.50*

1934 NURSING SCHOOL CLOSES. In an effort to consolidate expenses, the Alta Bates Board of Directors decides to close the nursing school. Some 330 nurses have graduated from the school in its 29 years. Some of those graduates will return to Alta Bates for their first reunion in October 1978, and the memories will flow. "We did a lot of things that aren't done now," Mrs. Hazelmae Wigmore Spainhower of Berkeley (Class of 1934) will recall on that occasion.

1934 Two new additions increase capacity at Herrick to 100 beds. William Walter Reich, MD, establishes a part-pay clinic to serve outpatients who can't afford private care and are ineligible for county or other forms of aid. Physicians donate services and the hospital uses a sliding scale fee system.

1934 The 2,100-acre East Bay Regional Park District is born; Wildcat Canyon (later called Tilden) is one of its first parks. (It will grow to 50,000 acres in Alameda County and 42,000 acres in Contra Costa County.)

1935

1935 Amelia Earhart lands in Oakland after the world's first solo airplane flight across the Pacific. This same year, the Social Security Act becomes law and Alcoholics Anonymous is founded.

1936 The first modern "miracle" drug, sulfanil-amide, drastically changes the treatment of pneumonia and peritonitis.

1936 Alta Bates files papers as a not-for-profit corporation. Among the purposes described in the Articles of Incorporation: "to establish, equip, maintain, operate, and conduct a hospital, dispensary, sanatorium or sanitoriums [sic] for the treatment and care of the sick, disabled, and infirm in the State of California." Bond holders return IOUs for little recompense as a donation to keep the hospital open.

It takes another 10 years for the hospital's reorganization as a not-for-profit institution to become official. A number of community leaders will join founder Miss Bates on the first Board of

Berkeley, 1931: Sales of poppies earn donations for needy World War I veterans.

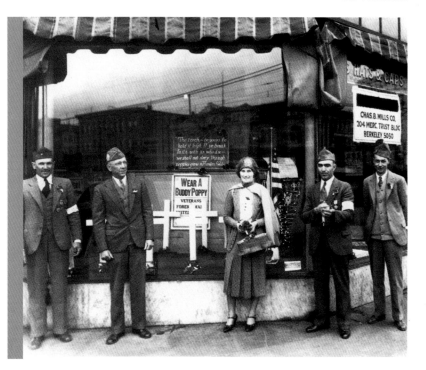

hard times hit home

It's a Depression-era tale that's often repeated: One evening, the story goes, retailer Lester Hink was visiting a friend in the hospital, when Miss Bates stopped by to greet him on her usual round of calls. Noticing that she looked exhausted, Hink asked her if she were ill. "No," she replied quietly. "But they're closing the hospital doors tomorrow."

In 1929, Alta Bates Hospital was facing bankruptcy. It was not alone. The country had just plunged into the Great Depression. Over the next few years, East Bay hospitals will fight for economic survival, as fewer patients will be able to pay for medical care—just when more people require it.

As it turned out, Alta Bates was rescued in large part by Hink, who owned a Berkeley department store. Hearing of the hospital's impending closure, Hink corralled 30 friends and colleagues, and in just one night raised $35,000 to keep the hospital doors open. Staying in the black is still dicey, so Alta Bates resorts to many cost-cutting measures. In 1930, salaries are slashed by 20 percent, reducing the average nurse's monthly wage from $150 to $120. In 1934, the nursing school is closed. For a while, the business manager, Gerrit Henry, even takes replaceable surgical blades to his local barber to have them sharpened for re-use!

When LeRoy Francis Herrick, MD, dies in 1932, the hospital he had founded (then called Berkeley General and later Herrick Memorial) is deep in debt and on the brink of closure. Herrick's granddaughter's husband, Alfred Maffly, a high school teacher and vice principal, takes over as the hospital's administrator. Maffly recognizes that the hospital cannot survive as a private, family-owned institution. He convinces Dr. Herrick's heirs to donate the hospital and reorganize it into a voluntary, not-for-profit, charitable organization controlled by a Board of Trustees.

Meanwhile in Oakland, Peralta Hospital administrators struggle to keep the facility afloat, with occupancy a scant 40 percent and two closed floors. When George U. Wood is named acting superintendent in 1933, the mortgage had not been paid for five years and the hospital is anticipating foreclosure. So Wood slashes room fees to raise the occupancy rate, initiates outpatient services, and in 1936, sees the hospital incorporated as a not-for-profit institution.

Providence, too, is hard hit by the Depression—not only because many patients can't pay, but because the hospital continues to fulfill its mission by serving 10,000–15,000 free meals a year. Through an innovative privatization program, Providence manages to continue its free meals and reduce its rates. In 1931 and 1932, the hospital leases its X-ray, cardiography, and pathology departments to private doctors.

Like many cash-strapped medical facilities across the country, East Bay hospitals labor mightily to stay financially solvent during the Great Depression. Only with the community's generous help and a dose of smart management do they survive the economic crisis, bolster themselves for the war years, and prosper in the better times to come.

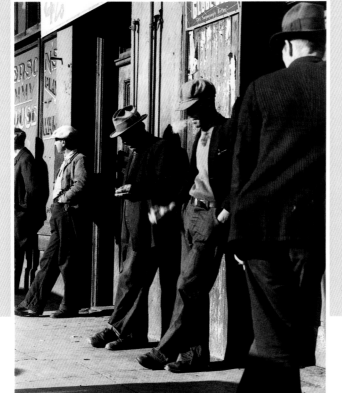

Bay Area men wait their turn in a bread line, a scene captured in the lens of famed Depression-era photographer Dorothea Lange.

40

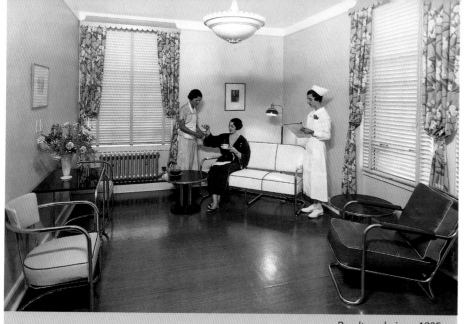

Peralta solarium, 1935

silent film entitled *Behind the Scenes in a Modern Hospital.* The color motion picture portrays day-to-day workings of a hospital, including a cesarean section procedure, and stars Peralta physicians, staff, and patients.

According to Wood's recollections, the film was an immediate success. Film rental fees supported the Peralta Hospital Endowment Fund, which aided premature babies and newborn babies needing extended hospitalization. Over the years, the film will be shown in medical schools throughout the world.

1936 Nancy Lee Vogt, about 15 ounces at birth and less than 12 inches long, is born two months premature on February 2 at Peralta. She makes headlines as the world's tiniest baby.

Peralta is swamped with mail from well-wishers—letters filled with prayers and home remedies—and the switchboard is besieged with calls. In the end, John Sherrick, MD, must sadly report that the baby was "doing unusually well" up to March 25, but took a downturn that day and died. Writes Dr. Sherrick, "Her death is explained by her immaturity with improper development and functioning of certain of her vital organs."

1936 BLUE CROSS COMES TO THE BAY AREA. Blue Cross is formed in the Assembly Room of Peralta. The innovative health organization is started by associates of Peralta, based on a concept that pioneered in Texas in 1929.

1937 Wood, Peralta's administrator, serves as producer, director, and cinematographer of a landmark

1937 Excerpts of an article published in the June *Bulletin of Peralta Hospital:*
"... The progress of surgical technique now has slowed down because operations and instruments

(continued on page 44)

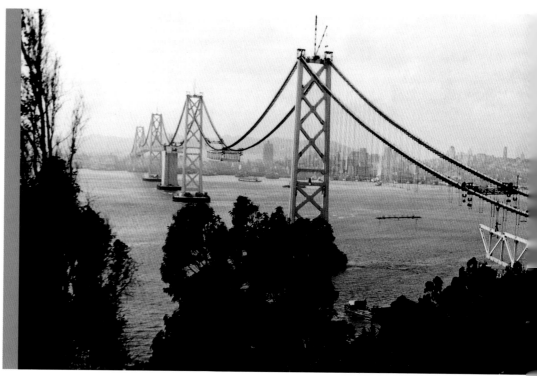

A spectacular view of the San Francisco-Oakland Bay Bridge under construction, before the decks are added. The span takes more than three years to complete and opens November 12, 1936. At this time, it is the world's longest steel bridge.

have become so perfected that only when highly specialized instruments are used in a small area of the body can we expect much change. ..... In conclusion, it may be stated that in the past 50 years surgery has made more progress in the preservation of human life than it had in the entire previous history of mankind."

1937 Scientists in the Soviet Union achieve success in producing the first vaccine to combat the troublesome human influenza virus. Magnetic resonance imaging—MRI—is developed in the United States by Isidor Rabi and Polykarp Kusch.

1937 MERRITT OPENS NEW WING. The three-story addition (with basement) north of the Administration Building will become known as the Ehmann Wing, in honor of its donors. (The Ehmanns had been inspired to make the gift after a lack of space forced their daughter to deliver her baby elsewhere.) The new wing includes six surgery rooms, a maternity department, patient rooms, and a clinical pathology lab. One newspaper's coverage of the opening, captioned "Pretty Soft for Babies," observes: "Life is easy for infants born in the new wing of Oakland's Merritt Hospital. The nursery, one of the most modern in the land, is air-conditioned. That makes it nice for nurses, too, who say the babies cry less. Fathers also get a break—the nursery is glass-enclosed, giving proud parents a fine view of their offspring."

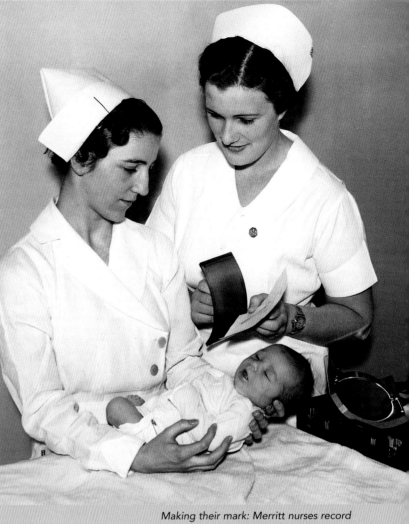

Making their mark: Merritt nurses record a newborn's footprint, 1936.

The need for larger, more modern quarters had become evident after Fabiola Hospital's closure in 1932. The wing is completed just in time. From a total of 872 babies delivered in 1938, yearly births at Merritt rocket to 2,242 by 1948.

1937 The Herrick Memorial Hospital Guild is founded, comprised of eight women who provide layettes and raise money for the hospital. This is the first organized fundraising program for a Berkeley hospital.

1937 Amelia Earhart's plane takes off from Oakland Municipal Airport and she begins her ill-fated flight around the world.

1937 Playwright Eugene O'Neill is presented his 1936 Nobel Prize medal for Literature while a patient at Merritt Hospital.

1938 The plastic contact lens is introduced by Theodore E. Obrig. Charles A. Poindexter and M. Bruger demonstrate the statistical significance of a high cholesterol level in heart disease.

1938 Occupational therapy is introduced at Merritt. The facility's endowment fund supports $6,500 of free hospital care.

This same year, a school for medical librarians is founded at the hospital. One graduate, Barbara Hastings, becomes the longtime secretary to the board of directors.

1938 PERALTA CELEBRATES ITS 10TH ANNIVERSARY. Exhibits at the anniversary festivities include the newest patient rooms, featuring bedside radios.

Dr. Sherrick, chairman of the day, remarks: "Since opening day, Peralta Hospital has grown in stature, in usefulness, and in the affections of the people, and has kept pace with the advances in the science of medicine and surgery; it has extended its services to some 36,700 patients, giving back full health or a modicum of good health to a large majority and with it the ability to live and to love and to laugh and to play and to work. [Some] 5,996 new babes have been launched upon their experience with life."

1939 Ernest Lawrence wins the Nobel Prize for Physics, UC Berkeley's first recipient. (During the '40s and '50s, seven faculty members at Cal receive Nobel Prizes.)

1939 Peralta patients are served coffee in special demitasse cups, complete with linen napkins, between early wake up and breakfast.

Even the most cantankerous patients cheer up with this routine, says Peralta Superintendent Wood. The practice has completely eliminated the complaints from guests about waiting for breakfast, and is considered a noteworthy innovation.

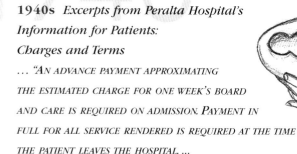

1940s *Excerpts from Peralta Hospital's Information for Patients:*
Charges and Terms
... *"AN ADVANCE PAYMENT APPROXIMATING THE ESTIMATED CHARGE FOR ONE WEEK'S BOARD AND CARE IS REQUIRED ON ADMISSION. PAYMENT IN FULL FOR ALL SERVICE RENDERED IS REQUIRED AT THE TIME THE PATIENT LEAVES THE HOSPITAL. ...*

It is the desire of the hospital to furnish good service. Criticisms and suggestions are solicited and should be made to the Superintendent. All communications should be addressed to the Superintendent."

Jazz is alive and well in Oakland in the 1930s.

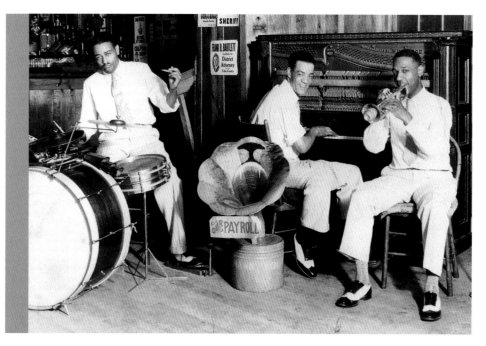

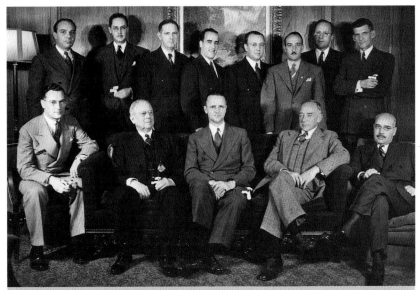

Eric Liljencrantz, MD, (bottom row, center) is the first member of Peralta's staff to be called for active military service, 1941.

1940s In the early years of this decade, the first kidney dialysis machine is developed.

1941 With the U.S. entrance into World War II looming, the Red Cross trains nurses' aides at Fairmount Hospital for the County of Alameda. One of these volunteer aides is Frances Hanna, who takes charge of the Berkeley nurses' aide program at Alta Bates.

1941 THE UNITED STATES ENTERS WORLD WAR II. On December 7, "a date which will live in infamy," Japanese forces stage a surprise attack on Pearl Harbor.

1941–1942 Within just a few months after America enters the war, the Defense Program and the resulting expansion of industries creates an alarming shortage of hospital beds in the Bay Area. The Oakland Hotel, once used for some festive social gatherings, conventions, and wealthy travelers, becomes a military hospital; in East Oakland, the Navy builds the Oak Knoll Naval Hospital. The federal government requests existing hospitals to do whatever is possible to increase bed capacity.

At Providence, the Sisters redesign some areas of the hospital and are able to increase capacity somewhat; despite these and other efforts, the acute demands continue to tax the hospital and its staff.

1941–1945 During the war years, Kaiser Shipways in Richmond, Calif., and Seattle, Wash., produces nearly 1,500 Liberty and Victory cargo ships, tankers, frigates, and sundry other vessels, according to a 2004 Oakland Museum of California exhibit. Innovative programs instituted by company founder Henry J. Kaiser, include a fledgling health care system for his workers. In 1942, Oakland's Permanente Foundation Hospital becomes the first of several Kaiser health plan hospitals.

1941–1950 Due to the influx of laborers for the war effort, Berkeley's population grows nearly 40 percent—from about 85,000 to 115,000. Oakland's population increases from 302,163 in 1940 to 400,935 in 1945.

The shipyards advertise nationally, recruiting thousands of women (some 25 percent of shipyard workers are females) and laborers of color with offers of high wages and immediate placement. However, blacks who apply at privately held plants confront whites-only hiring policies.

When the war ends, most of the migrants remain in the Bay Area. In Oakland, the black population grows from 8,462 in 1940 to 47,582 in 1950. Increasing numbers of Latinos, primarily people of Mexican origin, also come to the East Bay in the 1940s and 1950s.

THE WAY WE WERE

1940–1949:

U.S. population: 132,122,000

Berkeley population (1940): 85,547

Oakland population (1940): 302,163

Life expectancy: male, 60.8; female, 68.2

Average salary: $1,299/year

National debt: $43 billion

Minimum wage: $0.43/hour

55 percent of U.S. homes have indoor plumbing

Supreme Court affirms blacks' right to vote

World War II changes the order of world power; the United States and the USSR become superpowers

Cold War begins

Source: HandPrints, Children's Hospital Oakland

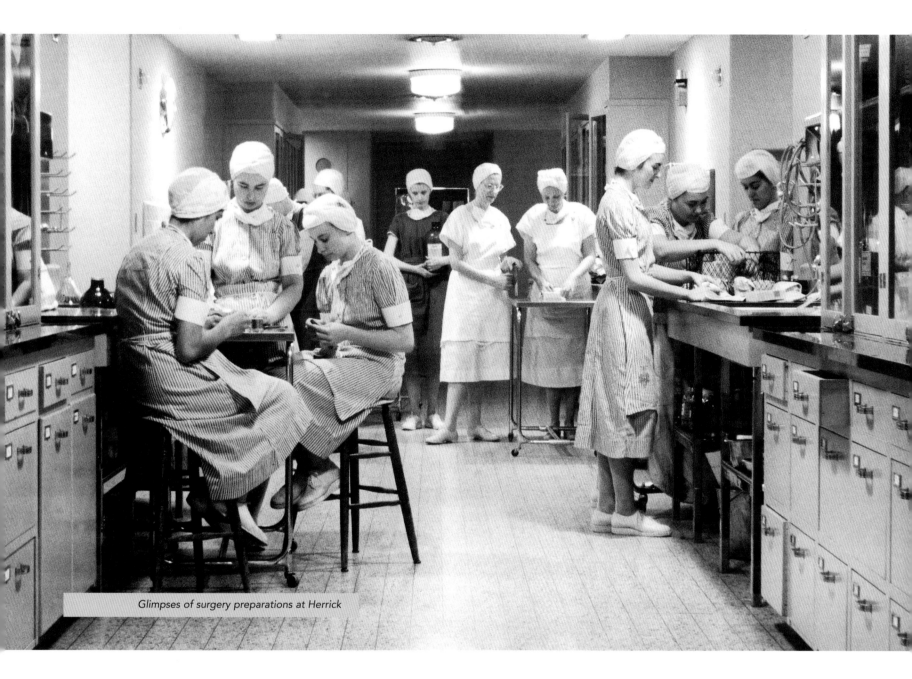

Glimpses of surgery preparations at Herrick

"In the past 50 years, surgery has made more progress in the preservation of human life than it had in the previous history of mankind." —*Bulletin of Peralta Hospital,* 1957

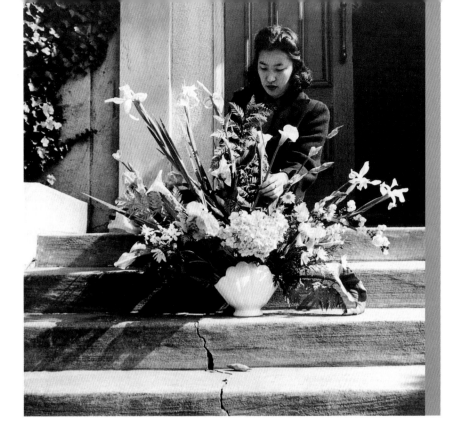

The hospital's census is high and beds in the corridor are a common sight.

1941–1945 On the community front, the focus is on conservation. Gasoline and food are rationed. Luxury items, such as silk stockings, are in extremely short supply. Rubber products, such as tires and even rubber bands, are used for the war effort. Families tend "victory gardens," where they grow their own vegetables so that as much food as possible can go to the troops. Children donate their metal toys, and the extra steel is used to help build ships.

1942 Discoveries by Daniel Bovet, a Swiss-born Italian pharmacologist, pave the way for treatment of human allergic conditions. H.D. Adams and L.V. Hands of Boston perform the first successful electrical defibrillation on a human.

1942 In Executive Order 9066, President Franklin D. Roosevelt authorizes the forced relocation and detention of 120,000 Japanese Americans as well as more than 2,000 Japanese Latin Americans. Tanforan Race Track in San Bruno is pressed into duty as an "alien assembly center."

Many internees, including some 12,000 Japanese Americans, respond to the War Department's 1943 call for volunteers to join an all-Japanese combat unit, the 442nd Regimental Combat Team. This legendary force will become the most decorated military unit in U.S. history.

1942 Excerpt from a May 27 newspaper clipping headlined, "Hospitals Here Set for Crisis":
Approximately 1000 hospital beds will be available at all times for the treatment of Oakland's civilian casualties in a war emergency.

This was disclosed last night by George U. Wood, chairman of the hospital committee of the Oakland Defense Council, as more than 375

Above: Arranging an altar bouquet at a Japanese church on the last day of services before evacuation and internment, 1942

Below: Latino workers at the Southern Pacific Railroad yard in Oakland, 1944

1941 Lake Merritt's 3,400-bulb "Necklace of Lights" (decorative illumination) goes dark when wartime blackout conditions are enforced.

1941–1945 During the war years, Peralta endures food and gas rationing, stringent priority ratings for hospital supplies, and wage and price controls. Doctors and nurses are needed for military service.

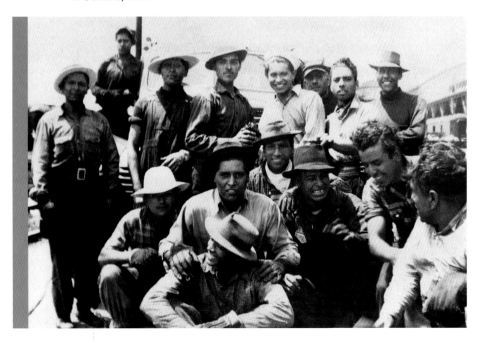

doctors and nurses gathered in Providence Hospital auditorium....

For several months, Wood said, Oakland hospitals have been extending their facilities to meet an emergency. Many thousands of dollars, he said, have been spent in preparing hospitals for all-night blackouts, installation of emergency units, and increasing inventories for necessary medical and surgical supplies.

1943 The U.S. Surgeon General announces allocation of funds to provide for the training of nurses under the newly founded Nurse Cadet Corps. Providence and Merritt participate.

1943 The transition between the Great Depression years and the accelerating demands of wartime tax Providence's resources and the Sisters' ingenuity to confront obstacles and respond to Oakland's changing needs. During 1936, 20 sisters maintain a staff of 59 employees and 74 nurses; they admit 3,421 patients. By 1943, 17 sisters maintain a staff of 120 employees and 219 nurses. The number of patients admitted triples to 9,653 in this year.

1943 Herrick receives $435,000 through the Lanaham Act for construction of the South Wing.

1943 The pap smear test is developed by G.N. Papanicolaou and H.F. Traut.

1944 Alta Bates' sale of stock to the community in the late '30s raised greatly needed capital. (The cost per share was 23 cents.) In 1944, the Board approves a two-cent dividend to stockholders "on each and every share of stock." Also, the Borden Company donates a refrigerator to be used in the new hospital Blood Bank, one of the most prominent philanthropic deeds recorded to this point.

1944 By this time, Alta Bates is in an improved financial position. In keeping up with new advances in medicine, the hospital upgrades its small X-ray and clinical laboratories into complete departments. After World War II, Henry Zwerling, MD, arrives, and a little later William Picard, MD. (In 1972, the medical staff will rename the Department of Diagnostic Radiology in honor of Dr. Zwerling.)

David Singman, MD, joins Alta Bates as a full-time pathologist in 1944. Until then, the small lab had operated with only a part-time pathologist (who also made the rounds of other hospitals in

building a tradition
1932–1949

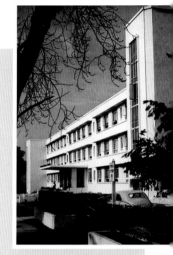

Herrick Memorial Hospital, 1949

HERRICK

1934 Two additions; capacity increases to 100 beds.

1945 Major facelift with modern, four-story main wing; capacity now totals 250 beds.

MERRITT

1932 Building and real estate acquired from newly closed Fabiola Hospital (property sold in 1942)

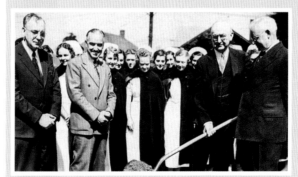

Groundbreaking ceremonies in honor of Merritt's Ehmann Wing

1937 Three-story addition (with basement), becomes known as the Ehmann Wing.

PERALTA

1949 New two-story wing built for $637,982; with furnishings and fixtures, the cost nears $1 million.

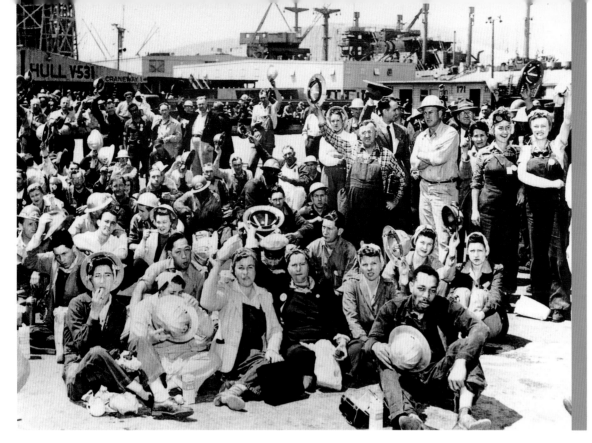

With women working shoulder to shoulder with men at Oakland's Moore shipyards, Rosie the Riveter's "We Can Do It!" credo comes to life, 1942.

1944 Herrick's Junior Volunteers program, founded by Mrs. B.T. Rocca, begins training enthusiastic Girl Scouts as hospital aides to help relieve the war-driven nursing shortage.

1944 The first TV sets hit the market. In Oakland, the Mai Tai drink is concocted at Trader Vic's.

1945 ALLIES CELEBRATE V-E DAY.
"Worst War in History Ends 3 P.M. Today," declares the *Berkeley Daily Gazette*'s May 8 front-page headline. The article boldly proclaims: "The bloodiest war in Europe's history ends officially at 6:01 p.m. EWT today with the unconditional surrender of Germany scheduled to be ratified in the ruins of Berlin."

1945 The day after V-E Day, Oakland voters demonstrate their optimism by approving more than $15 million in city improvement bonds, including monies for new playgrounds, swimming pools, libraries, streets and sewers, police, and courts.

1945 The United States drops atomic bombs from the skies over Hiroshima and Nagasaki. "The United

the area). From the start, Dr. Singman is an innovator. In this year, he establishes the Alameda County Blood Bank; later he will introduce new techniques—including computerization, for example—in the Alta Bates Laboratory. He dies following a heart attack in 1971, after 30 years as director of the Clinical Laboratory.

Medicine is just beginning to incorporate some of the new technology and treatments discovered during the war years, but is still far less sophisticated than it will be by the 2000s. The common procedures in '48 are hysterectomies, appendectomies, tonsillectomies, adenoidectomies and some vascular surgery—performed without the sophisticated medical equipment that will be available in the 21st century. Because of advances in administering anesthesia and in controlling infections, surgeries will be completed in the 2000s that weren't even considered possible in the '40s.

The Oakland Tribune *trumpets the war's end in Europe.*

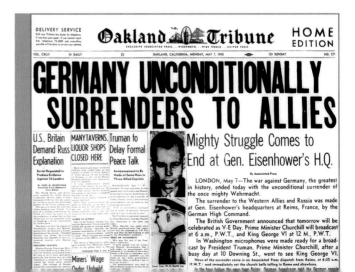

States has unleashed against Japan the terror of an atomic bomb 2,000 times more powerful than the biggest blockbusters ever used in warfare," Berkeley's *Gazette* reports. "President Truman revealed this great scientific achievement today and warned the Japanese that they now face a 'rain of ruin' from the air the like of which has never been seen on this earth."

1945 Representatives of 50 countries meet in San Francisco to draw up the United Nations Charter.

1945 President Roosevelt calls for selective service induction of nurses and the first proposal to draft women reaches the House of Representatives (unmarried graduate nurses, ages 20 to 44).

1945–1949 World War II sends University of California enrollments to all-time highs, and thus the population of Berkeley, and sets the stage for explosive suburban growth after the war. (In 1945, the *Berkeley Daily Gazette* reports Cal is the largest university in the nation.) The GI bill leads to increased enrollments, and postwar prosperity makes it possible for thousands to attend college. The campus now expands into surrounding residential neighborhoods.

Football will again be king as Cal plays in the Rose Bowl in the late 1940s and a new professional football team springs up across the Bay—the San Francisco 49ers.

1945 HERRICK GETS A FACELIFT. Berkeley General Hospital changes its name to Herrick Memorial Hospital and completes its modern, four-story main wing.

Capacity now totals 250 beds. "Berkeley Hospital Transforms Dream of Huge Medical Center Into Reality," declares a *Berkeley Daily Gazette* headline of the day.

Colleagues will later recall Dr. Walter Reich's inspirational comments at the wing's dedication: "We should pay tribute to the wonderful staff, the fine work of individual members, their interest, and devotion. But we should do that only in passing, for Herrick Memorial Hospital, the reality of a dream, is more than any one individual. It is a way of life!"

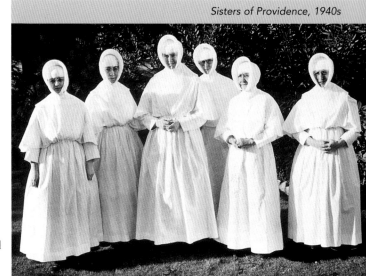

Sisters of Providence, 1940s

This same year, hospital trustees approve the Berkeley Council of Social Agencies' Inter-Racial [sic] Code and commit to accept patients, doctors, and staff without regard to race, religion, sex, age, or national origin.

1946 Cortisone is synthesized. This same year, Benjamin Spock, MD, publishes his groundbreaking book, *The Common Sense Book of Baby and Child Care.* (When Dr. Spock dies in 1998, his book will have been translated into 39 languages and sell more than 50 million copies, second in sales only to the Bible.)

1946 The Hill-Burton Act provides federal money to build hospitals across the United States, with stipulations for some free care to indigent patients. At least 9,200 buildings are raised.

1946 By the end of the war, Oakland is the 25th largest city in the nation. One fourth of all new industry in Northern California since the war began is located here.

1946 Oakland is introduced to Lee Susman's "Li'l Acorn." Through this popular cartoon character,

embracing diversity

When President Truman's Committee on Civil Rights issues its landmark 1947 report "To Secure These Rights," calling for an immediate end to "all discrimination and segregation based on race, color, creed, or national origin in ... all branches of the Armed Services," it signals an acceleration in social change that's fueled by the return of millions of World War II enlistees of every race and creed. In this era, the Berkeley Council of Social Agencies (reported in the 1945 *Berkeley Daily Gazette* as including the PTA, the city's Board of Education, and other groups) promotes its Inter-Racial Code for Social Agencies. Herrick's Board of Trustees adopts the code in 1945 and commits to an open-door policy for its patients, physicians, and staff. In subsequent years, Herrick will take

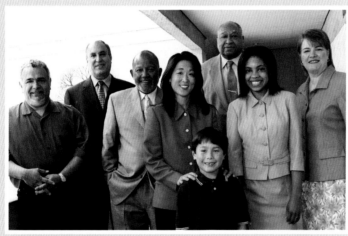

EHI team and supporters (left to right): Michael Carrillo, Vishu Lalchandani, Michael LeNoir, MD (EHI co-founder), Arlene Swinderman (Asian Outreach Program coordinator) and son Jake, Frank Staggers, MD (EHI co-founder), Samantha Floyd, and Brenda Rueda-Yamashita

a leadership role among area hospitals in diversifying its clientele and its medical staff and officers.

East Bay hospitals' institutional commitment to diversity will come to fruition in the late '90s and early 2000s. The Asian Outreach Program will focus on Mandarin and Cantonese translation at the Summit campus, telephone translations, Asian menu options, translated signage and forms, screenings, and distribution of health materials. The Ethnic Health Institute (EHI) will emphasize prevention and reduction of health disparities in cardiovascular disease and stroke, cancer, diabetes, and asthma. EHI will conduct free community-based health screenings, health fairs, and symposia for health providers. By 2004, EHI's Ethnic Health America Network (TV health magazine, radio talk show, and radio spots for African American radio outlets) will reach an audience of 10 million nationwide.

which appears in the *Oakland Tribune*, fans of the Oakland Oaks minor-league baseball team can watch the team's progress during the season. This same year, the short-lived West Coast Negro Baseball League's Larks earn a championship with 36 wins and just 12 losses. The Larks barnstorm the West and Mid-West, playing exhibition games until 1949. Lionel "Lefty" Wilson, the Larks' ace pitcher, later serves as Oakland's first black mayor, from 1977 to 1990.

1946 Alta Bates officially becomes Alta Bates Community Hospital. As a not-for-profit corporation governed by a Board of Trustees, all excess funds are reinvested in the buildings, equipment, and services. Former stockholders, most of whom are active medical staff, become full-voting Community Members. Thus, Alta Bates' governance lies chiefly in the hands of physicians, an uncommon practice among hospitals of the day.

1947 Suren H. Babington, MD, establishes the Department of Postgraduate Education at Herrick, and the facility becomes a teaching hospital for medical and surgical interns and residents. Subsequently, hundreds of young physicians graduate from the hospital's medical education program.

Herrick's teaching function assures the superiority of its care, but maintaining educational excellence is costly because few instructional programs directly produce revenue. The programs include administrative and psychiatric residencies; training in clinical psychology and coronary care; continuing postgraduate education programs for doctors and nurses and other health professionals; and training of licensed vocational nurses, medical records technicians, orderlies, psychiatric nursing students, pulmonary medicine technicians, respiratory therapists, X-ray technologists, social workers, and recreation therapists.

1948 Buses replace streetcars in Oakland.

**1948 PERALTA'S NEW WING GETS UNDER-
WAY.** Excerpts from the *Oakland Tribune*:
Peralta Hospital to Build New Wing to Cost $637,982
*A new two-story wing to cost $637,982 will be
constructed at Peralta Hospital, it was announced
today by George U. Wood, executive vice-president
of the hospital association.... It will house a new
X-ray department, deep therapy, clinical laboratories, physical therapy, a pharmacy, electrocardiol-
ogy, emergency suite, women's surgery ward and
administrative offices.... The structure will be of
steel-reinforced concrete and will be earthquake-
proof, according to the plans.*

*The new wing was made necessary, Wood
said, by the population increase in Oakland and
its growing need for hospital facilities.
"Recognizing our responsibility to the public, we
decided to go ahead right away."*

1948 A.E. Bennett, MD, founds the Department of
Psychiatry at Herrick, the first inpatient psychiatric

service in California—and one
of the first in the West—to be
integrated into a private community general hospital. In the
eight-bed facility, patients can
be treated near their homes,
families, and friends rather than
being transferred to distant
institutions. In 2004, the 122-
bed psychiatric service will be
the largest in a hospital of its
kind in the East Bay.

1948 The Oakland Oaks are vic-
torious in capturing the Pacific
Coast League pennant.

1948 The U.N. creates the
World Health Organization.

1949 KPFA hits the airwaves
as the country's first listener-
supported radio station.

**1949 NEW LEADERS TAKE
THE HELM AT ALTA BATES.** The years are
beginning to take their toll on Miss Bates, now 69
years old. She has devoted her entire life to the
hospital as a nurse, teacher, anesthetist, and inspirational leader. She tenders her resignation in
December 1945. Beginning in 1946, she turns over
some of her responsibilities to others. E.C. Pitcher
becomes president of the Board of Trustees. After
Pitcher passes away, Laverne H. Kibbe, a Berkeley
merchant, will serve as president from 1948 to
1950. John A. Wentworth, who once conducted the
business management of the hospital, becomes its
latest administrator.

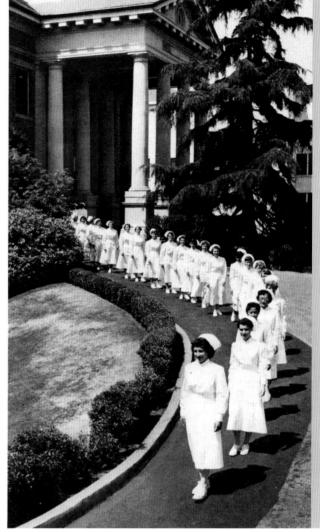

*One in a long line of
graduating classes
at Merritt, late 1940s*

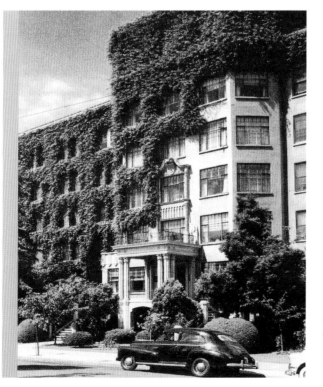

*Ivy bedecks exterior walls of Alta Bates;
operating rooms are on the top floor.*

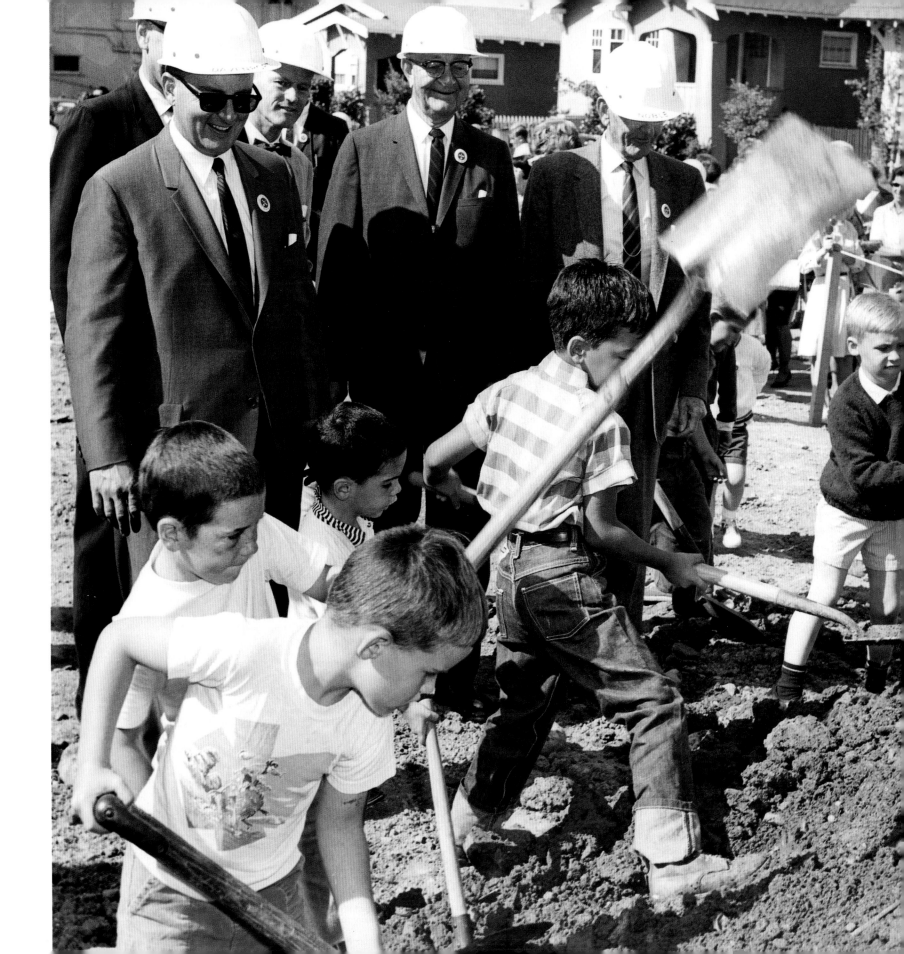

in peace and prosperity

Groundbreaking festivities in honor of Alta Bates Hospital's $6 million w

In the Bay Area as elsewhere, the 20th century's middle decades are times of explosive growth and social change. During the Civil Rights era, for example, Berkeley's school system integrates voluntarily while also initiating the nation's first non–court-ordered school busing plan.

Little wonder that the era's "can do" spirit is also reflected in East Bay medical facilities. Construction is the order of the day: From 1950 to 1979, Alta Bates, Herrick, Merritt, Peralta, and Providence hospitals boldly undertake 24 major capital projects. Given skyrocketing demand for their services, these facilities must rely more than ever on the ingenuity of their medical staffs and the untiring efforts of volunteers. Literally and figuratively, these institutions change the face of local health care.

Technology also continues to advance the hospitals' medical practice, pushed ahead by the Space Race that begins with the USSR's launch of Sputnik in 1957 and culminates a dozen years later with Neil Armstrong's—and mankind's—historic first steps on the moon. This period also sees, for the first time, open-heart surgery; the CT scan; liver, kidney, and heart transplants; amnio-centesis; and vaccines to safeguard against polio and measles.

Other landmarks include the mid-'60s debuts of Medicare and Medi-Cal. In the coming years, East Bay hospitals will feel the pinch as government continues to press for a health care safety net but fails to fully pay the bill. They'll be forced to consolidate their resources to meet evolving community needs.

1950

1950s As new types of general anesthesia are introduced in this decade, there is growing awareness that patients should be watched continually following surgery. After studying this need, Peralta Hospital opens a recovery room—the first in the country in a private medical facility. From the recovery room concept stems subsequent ideas for Peralta's first Intensive Care Unit in 1958 and its Coronary Care Unit in 1966.

1950s The Herrick Memorial Hospital Guild organizes into fundraising groups, inservice volunteers, and affiliated groups, to perfect a unique organizational structure, the "Crown of Jewels."

1950s Berkeley adopts its first master plan for the city, limiting population. The Berkeley Community Theater is built.

1951 The oral contraceptive (birth control pill) is formulated. It becomes available to consumers in 1960.

1951 This is a year of many changes for Alta Bates Hospital. The Board of Trustees amends the Articles of Incorporation, changing the name of the facility to Alta Bates Community Hospital and increasing the number of trustees from seven to 11 to broaden community representation.

Also this year, the hospital's namesake and founder leaves the East Bay to move to her summer home in Inverness. Miss Bates' adopted daughter, Peggy Bates Claussin, cares for her until she suffers a stroke and requires hospitalization. Marion Foster, RN, Miss Bates' "right arm" for many years, becomes the director of nurses and will serve for 35 years.

Foster is known as the "lady of the rose." In those days, "it was fashionable for nurses to wear fancy handkerchiefs in their breast pockets. But I always wore a fresh rose or camellia," Foster will later recall. In keeping with Miss Bates' tradition, she regularly visits each patient in the evening.

1951 Alta Bates is the East Bay's first community hospital to establish an isotope lab for diagnosis and treatment of human illness.

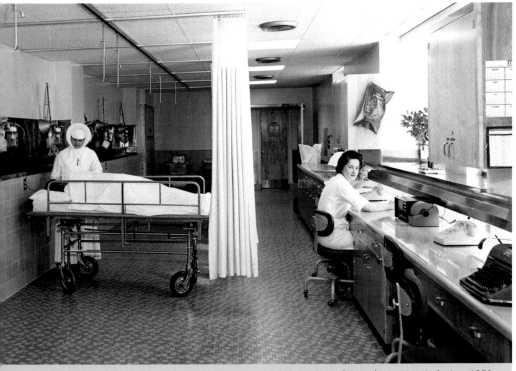

An insider's view of Providence Hospital, circa 1950s

1951 Now 47 years old, Herrick Memorial Hospital still has growing pains. To accommodate rapidly expanding services, the hospital's plant is enlarged as fast as it is financially possible. To keep step with its modern front, a project is begun to completely remodel the older sections of the building.

Also this year, Herrick debuts its electroencephalography program and is awarded $150,191 in Hill-Burton funds for the construction of the psychiatric inpatient unit.

1952 The first successful open-heart surgery is performed. The amniocentesis test is introduced.

1952 Oakland celebrates its centennial.

1952 ALTA BATES BEGINS FUNDRAISING.
As ambitious plans are being made for a new wing with 35 beds and new facilities for the hospital's laboratory, the Board of Trustees establishes a Permanent Building Fund to raise $450,000. Committees of interested citizens are organized to help inform the public of the community need and the reasons why voluntary hospitals require public support.

This is Alta Bates' first organized fundraising campaign. The physicians on staff respond with almost 100 percent participation. A donor can endow a four-bed room for $2,000; the Cradle Roll is established and requests donations honoring children born at Alta Bates. Over the years, handwritten names of Cradle Roll children will be displayed on hospital walls.

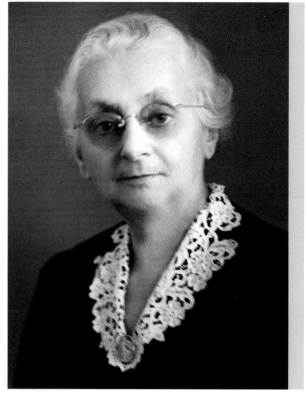

After nearly a half-century of dedicated service, hospital namesake and founder Alta Bates moves to her Inverness summer home in 1951.

1953 Watson and Crick describe DNA structure; the first link is revealed between diets high in animal fat and coronary heart disease; tests in mice suggest that cigarette tar may cause cancer; *Reader's Digest* magazine warns against smoking in its article "Cancer by the Carton."

1953 Alta Bates becomes the first hospital in the East Bay to establish a peacetime volunteer program, which is formalized as the Alta Bates Volunteer Association (ABVA) in 1956.

1953 The East Bay Rehabilitation Center (later Herrick's Department of Rehabilitation) is organized as the result of a study by the Oakland Community Welfare Council. In time, Herrick will have one of the largest and most extensive rehabilitation departments in the area.

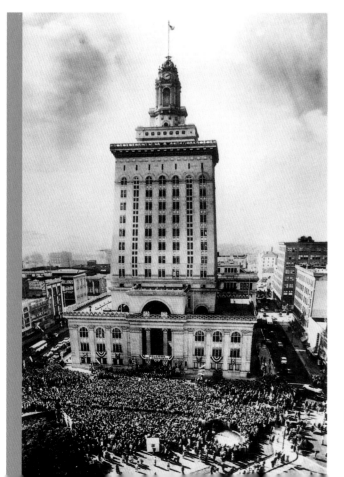

"We Like Ike": Crowds welcome President Eisenhower at Oakland's City Hall, 1952.

our crowning glory

Over the years, nurses' caps will fall out of fashion, but in earlier eras, this head gear holds more than mere eye appeal. Each nursing school has its distinctive style, donned proudly by its grads (including these Alta Bates nurses below).

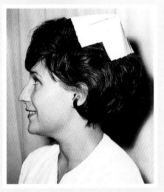

Jane Girard
University of Arizona

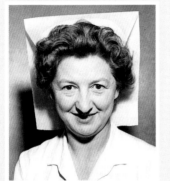

Frances Rath
Crumpsall Hospital, England

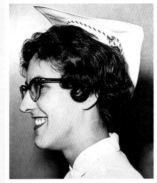

Gladys Grossini
University of California Hospital

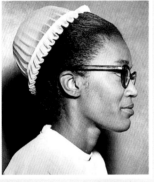

Ethel Jellins
Bellevue Hospital, New York

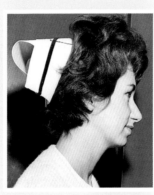

Florence Odegard
Saskatoon City Hospital, Canada

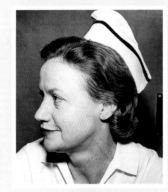

Regina Walsh
DePaul School of Nursing, St. Louis

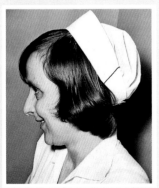

Rosle Roth
Schweiz-Pflegerinnen Schule, Zurich

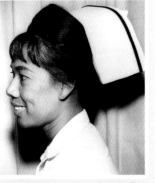

Pirkko Bentel
Etela-Saimaan
Sairaanhoitajakoulu, Finland

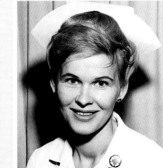

Joan Bermudez
St. Francis School of Nursing, Honolulu

1953 POLIO IS VANQUISHED. Jonas Salk, MD, reports findings on his discovery—the polio vaccine. The first successful human kidney transplant is performed and American scientists develop an implantable pacemaker, using the semiconductor transistor.

1954 ALTA BATES CELEBRATES ITS 50TH ANNIVERSARY. A block party in July on Regent Street, complete with balloons, ice cream, and displays on current hospital services, honors the founding of Alta Bates 50 years before. In November, the hospital officially dedicates the first phase of its new wing, erected on the original building's west side, with special ceremonies that take place at the site of what will be the new Physical Therapy Department and Clinical Laboratory. The unit adds 33 new beds.

1954 SCHOOLS DESEGREGATE. U.S. Supreme Court rules in landmark Brown v. Board of Education schools desegregation case.

1954 HERRICK IS 50. Herrick records the birth of approximately 75,000 babies in Berkeley during its first 50 years.

1955 ALTA ALICE MINER BATES DIES. The *Berkeley Daily Gazette* (December 1) reports:

Miss Alta A.M. Bates, founder of Berkeley's Alta Bates Community Hospital, was mourned today. She died at 5:30 p.m. Wednesday after an illness of more than two years. She was 76.

At the time of her death, Miss Bates was at a nursing home directly across the street from the hospital she founded. The home is operated by Miss Gertrude Trezona, a member of the first graduating class of Miss Bates' old nursing school….

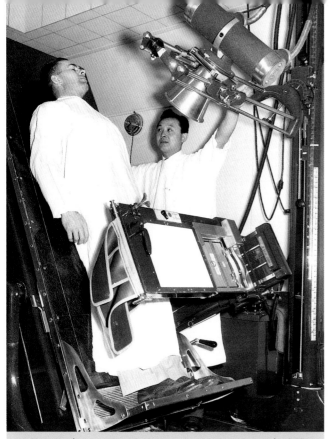

X-ray technician Kay Mori sets up at Merritt Hospital, 1952.

For many years before her retirement, Miss Bates was the hospital's chief anesthetist and one of the first women in the area proficient in that skill.

Even after her active association with the hospital ended, Miss Bates was a frequent visitor to patients at the hospital and her calls are remembered by many patients as a highlight of their hospital stay....

Advised of Miss Bates' death, Raymond M. Young, president of the hospital's board of trustees, said, "It was with the greatest sadness that I learned of Miss Bates' passing. None who knew her could help but be inspired by her great compassion for the thousands of afflicted persons who came to her hospital for care and attention. Her life-long dedication to the highest possible standards of nursing and medical care has been an influence more significant than many people realize, in the high quality of medical care available in our community. Her courageous,

pioneering spirit, together with her qualities and kindness and gentleness, constitutes a lasting tradition that will always be part of the hospital she brought into being."

1955 HERRICK INNOVATES. The hospital opens a part-pay psychiatric clinic for outpatients. Also in the '50s, Herrick becomes one of the first secular hospitals in the area to provide the services of a full-time hospital chaplain, who offers spiritual and emotional support to any patient who desires such help. Herrick also starts an inservice internship program in clinical pastoral care for seminary students and pastors.

1956 Some 71 percent of Alta Bates' 7,425 patients have hospitalization insurance of some sort—an increase of 10 percent over 1955, 16 percent higher than in 1951, and a sign of changing times in health care finance. The average stay of patients at the facility is 6.1 days.

1956 PROVIDENCE HOSPITAL ERECTS NEW WING. Providence's 1926 building is inadequate for the growth Oakland has experienced since the '40s, so expansion again becomes a priority on the Sisters' agenda. A new wing facing Webster Street is built. All offices are moved out of the main hospital and into the new wing to make room for more services and a 230-bed capacity.

1957 The first members of the Merritt Hospital Auxiliary are recruited. Later their motto will be: "We Must Keep Our Standards High."

facts and figures
1934-1954
HERRICK HOSPITAL

Surgical Operations

Year	Operations
1934	540
1939	818
1944	1,653
1949	4,216
1954	5,163

Pediatric Admissions

Year	Admissions
1934	1,385
1939	2,022
1944	4,716
1949	8,449
1954	8,917

Enchilada Shop owner Dominguita Velasco (second row left) poses with three generations of her family, including her daughter Rosita (front right), mother, sister, and niece, Oakland, 1955.

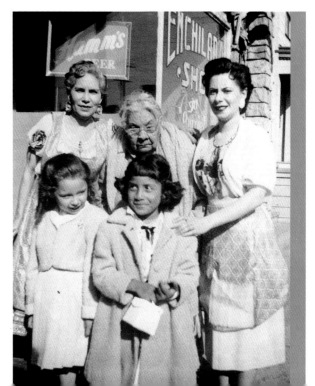

1957 MERRITT HOSPITAL BUILDS NEW WING. Merritt completes its Cobalt Wing, providing Northern California's first Teletherapy Unit for the treatment of cancer. The project costs $150,000 (two-thirds of the funding is raised through private funds and more than 500 donors). The addition can accommodate two Cobalt Units, the second installed in February 1961 at a cost of $110,000.

1957 HERRICK ADDS NORTH WING. Herrick adds a seven-story North Wing, which includes space for 49 psychiatric beds and an entire floor for rehabilitation facilities. Bed capacity reaches 287. "Today's hospital must care for the sick, but it must do more than that," says administrator Alfred Maffly. "It must carry on all four functions through which a modern hospital fully serves its community: patient care, public health, research, and education."

1958 Peralta opens the first surgical Intensive Care Unit (ICU) in the East Bay and the first

Radiation Therapy Unit in the Bay Area. The equipment includes a Maxitron for radiation treatments.

Herrick will be the first community general hospital in the East Bay to develop such a unit, which becomes a Surgical Intensive Care Unit in 1968. Merritt and Providence open ICUs in 1959–1960.

1959 Merritt agrees to accept credit cards from Bank of America and First Western Bank as payment for services.

1960s TURMOIL ROILS THE BAY AREA. The '60s bring revolutionary change to society. In 1962, California becomes the Union's most populous state, creating unprecedented demand for health services.

The decade also witnesses great social upheaval and political turmoil, sparked by rebellion of the young and the disadvantaged and highlighted by the local People's Park protests, Summer of Love, Peace and Freedom movement, and more. In these years, Cesar Chavez leads farm workers in a strike against California grape growers, galvanizing nationwide support.

1960 The Raiders come to Oakland in the new, and much ballyhooed, American Football League.

1960 New $390,000 outpatient facilities (a ground-floor addition) are constructed at Merritt. Merritt Hospital Volunteers form a Junior Auxiliary. Barbara B. Davies, graduate of Merritt School of Nursing, becomes the first female member

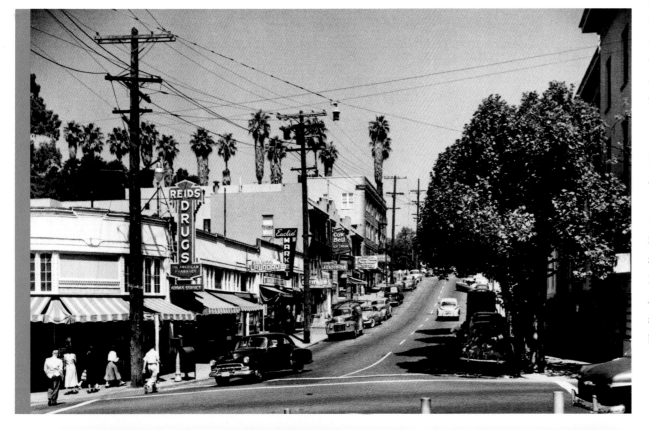

A slice of life on Berkeley's Euclid Avenue, 1959

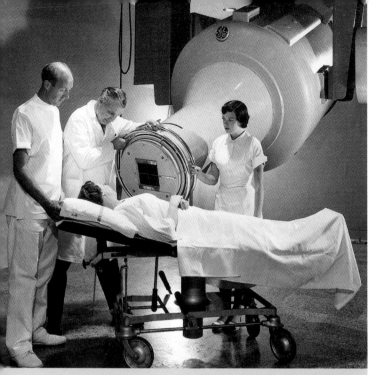

X-ray therapy at Peralta Hospital, 1958

of the Merritt Hospital Board of Directors, which increases from seven to 15 members.

1960 PILL HILL ZONED. The City of Oakland establishes a Medical Center District in the Pill Hill Area, and sets plans in motion to develop the 77-acre area into a complete medical center. The zoning designation reserves the major portion of the hill—home of Merritt, Providence, and Peralta—for uses directly related to medical treatment and research.

1961 Oakland's cargo tonnage grows dramatically as the first container ships dock at its harbor.

1961 Oakland City College begins a nursing program to combat a severe personnel shortage; Peralta is among the local hospitals assisting.

1961 Under the direction of Ivan May, MD, doctors perform the East Bay's first open-heart bypass surgery at Merritt's $35,000 coronary bypass center.

1962 Measles vaccine is developed by American Nobel Prize winner John Franklin Enders. The use of lasers in medicine becomes possible with Frenchman Marcel Bessis's invention of the microlaser.

1963 JFK KILLED. ACTIVISTS MARCH. The November 22 assassination of President John F. Kennedy rocks the nation and millions mourn his loss. Still fresh in Americans' memories is the August 28, 1963 March on Washington, D.C., which marks a high point in the civil rights movement with Dr. Martin Luther King Jr.'s "I Have a Dream" address before a crowd of more than 200,000.

1963 Herrick becomes the first community general hospital in the Bay Area to establish a Social Service Department. Here, trained professionals counsel patients and families about illness, disability or dependence, and help to relieve any anxieties that might hinder a patient's recovery.

(continued on page 64)

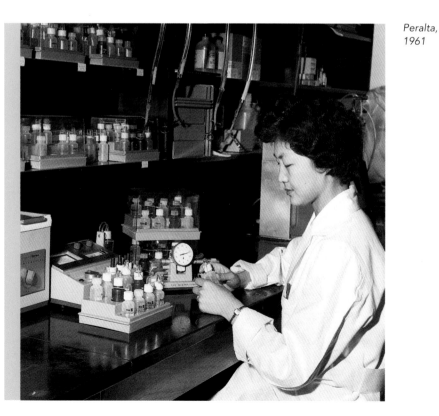

Peralta, 1961

helping hands

The contributions of volunteer groups at Providence, Alta Bates, Herrick, Merritt, and Peralta have been nothing short of remarkable. Over 100-plus years, volunteers have welcomed visitors, assembled patient charts, knitted booties, stuffed envelopes, shuttled absentee ballots during elections, hosted teas, sold thrift-store bargains, decorated the hospitals for the holidays, delivered lab tests, and cuddled preemies. As an observer once remarked: "These ladies could be running the country."

In the postwar period, for example, volunteers' fundraising and assistance in the hospitals blossom, energized by hospital auxiliaries' popularity. (Across the country, there are more than 1,500 of such groups in 1956 with combined membership of 500,000.)

Herrick Memorial Hospital Guild is revitalized in the '50s with the popular Crown of Jewels. Its many "arches," each named after a precious gem, unite volunteers toward particular goals, including fundraising and public relations aims. The Providence Hospital Auxiliary mirrors such division of labor with nine branches, each named for a California mission. Not all groups follow this model: In 1957, Merritt Hospital Auxiliary's charter members, including wives of staff doctors, nursing alumnae, and community friends, set their sights strictly on service.

Formal programs inside hospitals also spread in the '50s. At Peralta, crews run a gift shop that is the toast of the town—doctors' wives make a point to shop the stylish collection. At Merritt, enthusiasts provide coffee cart service. The Board of Trustees approves bylaws for the new Alta Bates Volunteer Association

in 1956, which expands earlier efforts by the Alta Bates Associates, an energetic group of doctors' wives that had joined forces to help refurbish the hospital. Herrick's first Volunteer Service director assumes the post in 1954.

Volunteers in this era are particularly adept at fundraising luncheons, fashion shows, gift sales, and gala social gatherings, including Herrick's ever popular Holiday Fair and Alta Bates' annual Red and White Ball (begun in 1957) and Evening of Elegance (the first in 1976). One notable twist on the conventional tea is Herrick's Operation Coffee Cup, held on May 6, 1954. That day, mugs of java are sold in a chain of fundraising coffee klatches throughout Berkeley. A later variation on the usual monetary solicitation: In 1971, Campfire Girls collect 1,200 Betty Crocker boxtop coupons, part of a drive led by Delta Zeta Sorority, a Herrick guild affiliate,

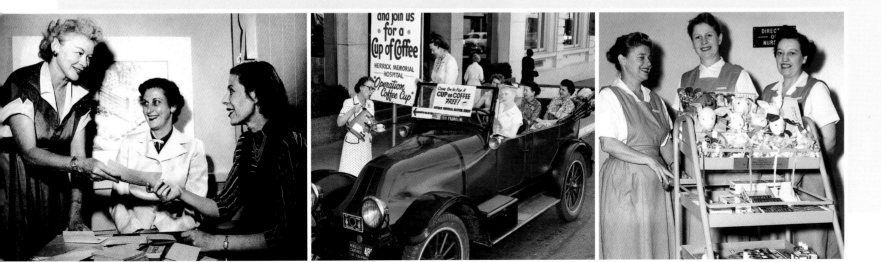

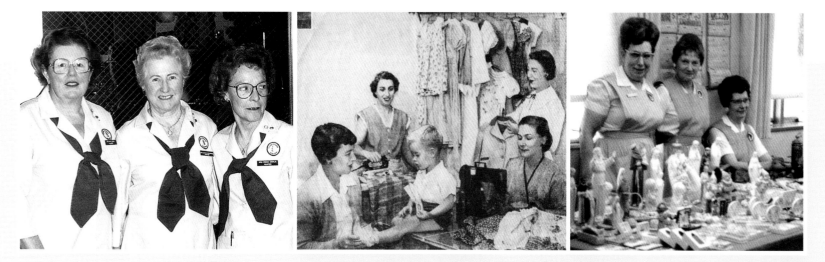

to redeem 720,000 coupons from General Mills for cash to buy an audiometer.

Volunteers are also experts at filling gaps in hospital resources and augmenting patient services in a variety of areas. Some examples: Alta Bates Foundation Associates' purchase of equipment for the new Burn Center in the mid-'70s; Herrick's award-winning Tele-Care program that begins placing daily calls to shut-ins in 1970 (and will continue to do so in the 2000s).

To be sure, the various postwar volunteer efforts draw on a longstanding tradition that consistently brought residents in the area, especially conscientious females, to their hospitals' aid. The Providence Hospital Auxiliary, for example, was founded in 1902, when a group of women gathered in one of the co-founders' homes, elected officers, and assessed themselves $.25 monthly dues. This group played a significant role in fundraising that assisted in founding Providence, the establishment of a part-pay children's clinic, and more.

Volunteers have made a crucial difference in times of crisis, as well. During World War II, for example, thousands of Red Cross nurses' aides helped remedy

East Bay hospitals' severe nursing shortage. Alta Bates' program, run by Frances Hanna (then Frances Hills), was a nationally recognized model. At Herrick, Girl Scouts served as junior nurses' aides.

In every era, volunteers have brought creativity to their charge. In the 1980s, Alta Bates Foundation Associates' one-day "Hook a Million" giveaway will promise $1 million to whomever can snag a specially tagged leopard shark from the San Francisco Bay. (No winner!) Also in the '80s, Alta Bates volunteers begin nationwide sales of hospital uniforms, netting more than $1 million by 2004.

In the early 2000s, the volunteer spirit will still be alive and well. Alta Bates Summit Volunteers will log 47,376 volunteer hours in 2003. Alta Bates Summit Associates' thrift store, "The Showcase," will pass the $3 million mark in its fundraising. Providence Auxiliary will operate the Summit Campus' two gifts shops. "People become volunteers for a variety of reasons," says Thora Loutfi, Alta Bates Summit's director of volunteer development and services. "But what I've heard them say again and again over the years is that they get more out of it than they put in."

Opposite, left to right:
Doctors' wives prepare for their next fundraiser.
Dollars pour in for a one-of-a-kind Herrick fundraiser.
Merritt's Courtesy Cart debuts, 1957; left to right: Mrs. Michael Neff, Mrs. Ernest Romine, and Mrs. Paul Lofholm.

Above, left to right: Peralta gift shop volunteers Providence's Carmel group outfits needy children, 1954. Gamelin Association volunteers survey the goods at a Providence bazaar, circa 1960s.

Below: Eager Candy Stripers at Alta Bates Alta Bates Summit gift shop volunteers, circa 2000s; left to right: Nancy Smith, Elizabeth Garner, and Helga Tannenbaum

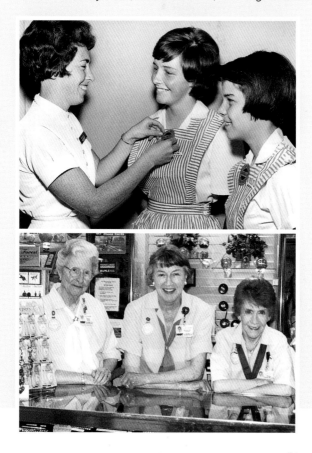

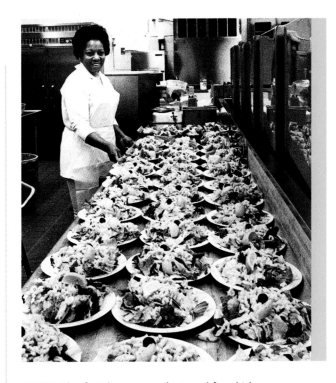

Alta Bates food service worker Velma Thomas executes mass production with a personal touch, 1967.

1963 The first liver transplant and first kidney transplant are performed. In 1967, the first heart transplant takes place in South Africa.

1963 The Nuclear Medicine Laboratory at Merritt opens for business.

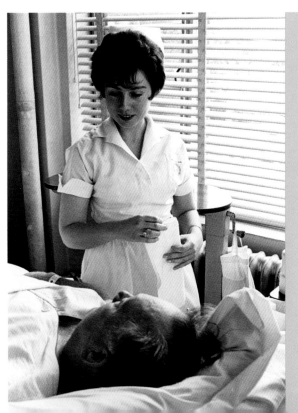

A Providence nursing student undergoes clinical training, circa 1960s. Economic shortfalls force closure of Providence's College of Nursing in 1972.

1964 PROVIDENCE GROWS. Providence adds a sixth floor to increase bed capacity. The expansion is followed by the debut of a Respiratory Care Unit in 1967, a Coronary Care Unit in 1968, and a Hemodialysis Unit in 1969. The following year a Hemodialysis Home Training Center with two beds is established at doctors' request. In 1970, the Sisters formally open a Nuclear Medicine Department, the Cerebro-Vascular Disease Unit and Employee Health Services. A year later, they start a 24-hour Emergency Service.

1964 MERRITT TOWERS. Merritt's new $4.5 million Central Tower adds 150 patient beds in "attractively decorated rooms offering electronic push-button services."

A fundraising brochure of the day describes the hospital's overburdened capacity: "Samuel Merritt Hospital carries a tremendous load. Each year it has nearly 10,000 patients, and its occupancy rate has exceeded the 80 percent level for the past several years. Often, occupancy has exceeded capacity."

Between 1954 and 1964, there have been dramatic increases in demands on the hospital. The number of emergency patients treated rose 84.6 percent to 4,250; outpatient visits increased 135.7 percent to 55,986; X-ray procedures were up 44.9 percent to 22,797.

1965

1965 Merritt celebrates its 56th anniversary with the announcement of Project 70, an $8 million expansion program that will make the hospital one of the nation's leading medical facilities.

The five-year program begins with a new school of nursing and student nurse residence to replace Farrelly Hall. The lower level classrooms surrounding Towne Court are a memorial to Mr. and Mrs. George S. Towne, contributed by their children. Completion of the new educational facility in 1966 is marked by a homecoming for more than 1,000 of the school's graduates. The student residence is christened Bechtel Hall, in honor of Stephen D. Bechtel, a major contributor to the building project.

1965 HERRICK EXPANDS. A four-story auditorium and clinic building is added, along with a chapel, radioisotope laboratory, and an entire floor for psychiatric outpatient care. The Pulmonary Function Laboratory is initiated.

In the following year, electromyography is provided and the Radioisotope Laboratory opens.

1965 Peralta, which now boasts 205 licensed beds, witnesses its first on-site wedding, fulfilling an ailing patient's wish to witness her son's rites. The *Oakland Tribune* headlines its April 15 report, "Hospital Nuptial Knockout Event."

1965–1966 MEDICARE AND MEDI-CAL ARE BORN.

National health insurance for the aged—Medicare—becomes effective on July 1, under Title 18 of the 1965 Amendments to the Social Security Act. Following suit, California establishes the Medi-Cal program and essentially gives all Californians drawing welfare compensation access to medical care in any qualifying hospital.

1966–1968 ALTA BATES ERECTS NEW WING.

Alta Bates constructs a new $6 million, six-story wing to house 52 new beds, a new surgical suite; Clinical Laboratory; diagnostic X-ray; electroencephalography, electromyography, electrocardiology, and radioisotope services; physical and radiation therapies; Emergency Outpatient Department; engineering; and laundry.

The campaign had received a boost with major contributions in memory of two of the hospital's prominent leaders: a gift of $294,000 from the estate of Raymond M. Young and a gift of $1 million from the estate of C. Mahlon Kline in memory of his nephew Mahlon Kline Jordan.

In tribute to these two loyal supporters, the hospital will dedicate the new wing to Young in 1968 and the Acute Care Center to Jordan.

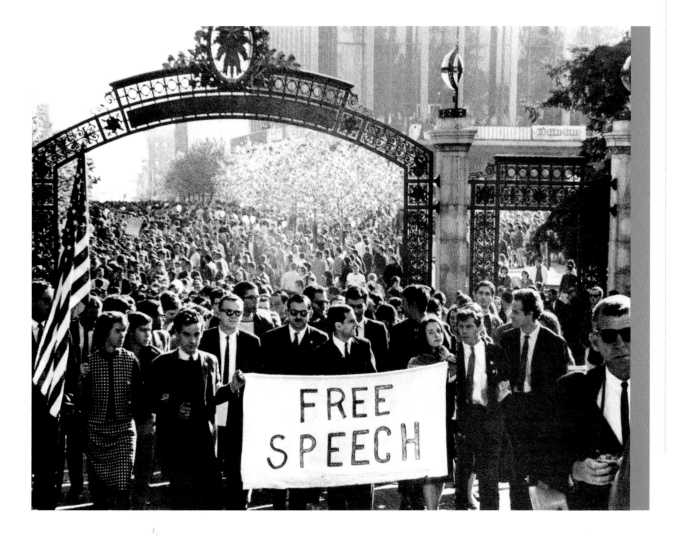

Mario Savio leads the University of California's Free Speech Movement in 1964, sparking massive student demonstrations on the Berkeley campus and giving rise to campus sit-ins. Student protests at Cal date back to 1873; an antiwar movement was alive and well there before the U.S. entry into World War II.

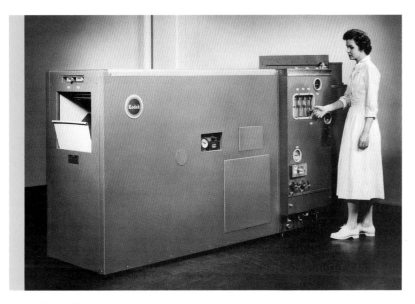

One of the first X-ray film processors, Peralta

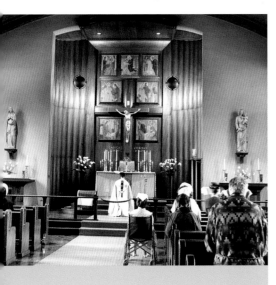

Benediction of the Blessed Sacrament, Providence Chapel (early 1960s)

Just prior to the dedication, John Peterson, who worked so hard to see the 1954, 1959, and 1968 building projects successfully completed during his service as administrator, resigns from Alta Bates. Robert L. Montgomery, who joined the hospital in 1963, assumes the post.

1967 John F. Wight succeeds Maffly as administrator at Herrick. Early this year, the hospital retains the architectural firm of Rex Whitaker Allen and Associates to assist in a master plan that will help the hospital meet the area's future health needs.

Berkeley's two community hospitals, Alta Bates and Herrick, recognize the need for joint planning. Representatives of the Boards of Trustees, medical staffs, and administrations of the two hospitals meet to discuss how they can best prepare for the challenging future.

1967 Herrick's Maternity Department closes and combines its services with Alta Bates. Herrick had been the first hospital in the area to institute rooming for mother and baby and to permit fathers in the delivery room during a birth.

1967 Providence introduces its Respiratory Care program. In this same year, Barbara Lynn Wicket is the 45,000th infant born at Merritt.

1967 A *Merritt Monogram* report details a troubling nursing shortage, which first surfaced shortly after World War II, and forecasts an even more critical shortfall.

1967 The Peralta Hospital Medical Foundation is formed, with retired Superintendent George Wood as its president.

1967 MERRITT COMPLETES PROJECT 70. In the second phase of Merritt's Project 70, a $1,700,000 wing for ancillary services opens.

The ambitious, long-range project will finally be completed in April 1971, with the opening of the new West Tower (bringing capacity to 350 beds) and a parking garage for 300 autos. The last of the hospital's original buildings, the old South Wing, will be removed in 1972 to give Merritt a sparkling new look.

Still other facets of Project 70 include the modernization of existing buildings for the addition of specialized equipment used in diagnostic

building a tradition

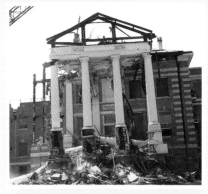

Merritt's South Wing comes down, 1972

MERRITT

1952 Merritt laboratory and X-ray departments move into 34th Street Wing, which was added to the Ehmann Wing.

1957 New Cobalt Wing

1960 New $390,000 outpatient facilities (a ground-floor addition)

1964 $4.5 million Central Tower adds 150 patient beds.

1966 New school of nursing and student nurse residence

1967 $1,700,000 wing for ancillary services

1971 New West Tower (bringing capacity to 350 beds) and parking garage for 300 autos

1972 Removal of the old South Wing, the last of the hospital's original buildings

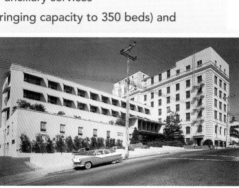

ALTA BATES

1954 New wing on the original building's west side adds 33 new beds.

1966–1968 New $6 million, six-story Raymond Young Wing houses 52 new beds, a new surgical suite, clinical laboratory, several departments, engineering, and laundry

1975 A new $17 million wing is built. Brand new beds are purchased for the 1928 building, and total bed capacity reaches 311.

HERRICK

1951 Older sections of the building are completely remodeled.

1957 New seven-story North Wing; bed capacity reaches 287

1958 Large addition—new patient rooms, new dining room, administrative wing, and more

1965 Clinic building added, plus four-story auditorium, chapel, radioisotope laboratory, and an entire floor for psychiatric outpatient care

1977 New five-story, 153-bed patient care wing replaces older facilities and adjoins the existing North Wing; construction cost is $9.8 million.

PERALTA

1950, 1954 Beds added; surgery and delivery rooms are remodeled.

1966 West Wing renovated

1978 Three-level Outpatient Services Building (43,000 square feet) is erected. Sherrick Building is dedicated.

Peralta

PROVIDENCE

1956 New wing facing Webster Street; 230-bed capacity

1964 Sixth floor is added; increases bed capacity.

1979 The new $22.5 million, 230-bed hospital opens, with four-story nursing wing and an additional wing for special-care inpatients.

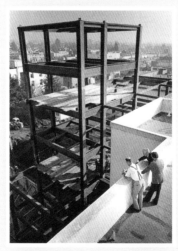

Herrick

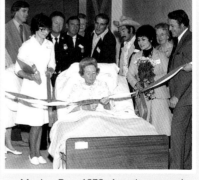

Moving Day, 1979: A patient cuts the ribbon to open the new Providence.

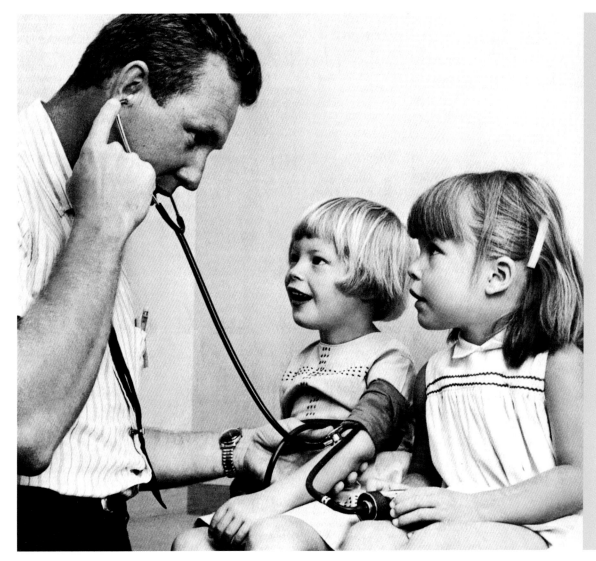

An Alta Bates physician engages fledgling patients in their care, 1966.

1968 The Bay Area's first total hip-replacement surgery is performed at Merritt by orthopedic surgeon William Jackson, MD. The hospital is one of only 20 medical facilities in the country originally licensed by the FDA to evaluate joint replacement. By the end of 1979, approximately 1,500 total hip-replacement procedures will be performed.

1968 Both Providence and Merritt open Coronary Care Units.

1968 Herrick devotes the clinic building's entire fourth floor to the new Acute Care Wing, with five private acute coronary care rooms, bringing the total number of acute care beds to 24 and the hospital's total bed capacity to 241. Respiratory therapy begins.

1969 Taking "one small step for man, one giant leap for mankind" on July 20, astronaut Neil Armstrong becomes the first man to walk on the moon.

1969 A hepatitis vaccine is introduced by American biochemist Baruch Samuel Blumberg.

and research work. This phase includes the $250,000 Cardiovascular Special Procedures Center made possible by an initial $100,000 contribution from the Alameda County Heart Association.

1968 CIVIL RIGHTS LEADER AND POLITICIAN ARE SLAIN. Just two months separate the shocking killings of civil rights activist Dr. King and Senator Robert Kennedy.

1968 The A's move from Kansas City to their new home in Oakland.

1960s–1970s The phenomenon of fewer Sisters of Providence in the Sacred Heart Province requires the hiring of lay administrators in the system. Providence's original Articles of Incorporation, which five sisters created in 1903, is amended to include all the Sisters' institutions in California. The lay administrators, professionals in the health care industry, manage the hospital in concert with and under the guidance of the Provincial House. The basic mission remains intact.

1970s Warren Widener is elected the first African American mayor of Berkeley.

The era of initiatives, preservation ordinances, and master plans reaches a high point in the city. Developments in programs for people with disabilities make Berkeley a trailblazer for the physically challenged.

1970s ALTA BATES FOUNDATION DEBUTS. By this time, state regulations concerning earthquake safety in hospitals have made the 1928 building unsuitable for inpatient care. Alta Bates' Board makes plans to locate most inpatient services in a relocated and expanded facility adjoining the hospital to the north.

In preparation for the major fundraising effort that will be necessary, the Board changes the Development Committee's name to the Alta Bates Foundation. Morris Doyle—"A strong man and instrumental in helping us raise money," according to Foundation Trustee Langfield—and Winifred Heard, a prominent civic and international leader, are most responsible for launching the Foundation.

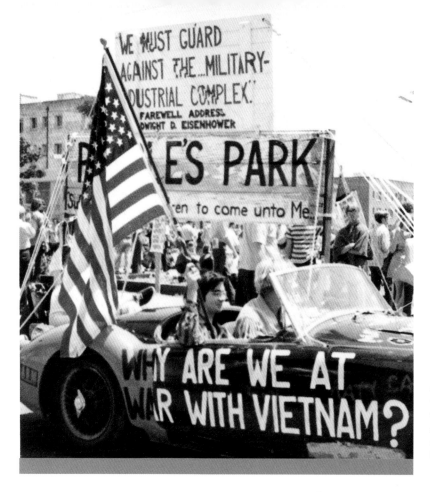

Berkeley is in the forefront of the 1960s anti-war and anti-establishment activism.

1970 Herrick's Angioplasty and Cardiovascular Laboratory open. The new Pastoral Counseling Service provides professional counseling to residents of Berkeley and surrounding areas. In this decade, Herrick collaborates with Alta Bates to establish the Cardiac Rehabilitation Program at the YMCA, one of the first of its kind in the Bay Area.

1970 Herrick's Tele-Care Program, one of the nation's original telephone reassurance programs, begins. The program will win several awards, including recognition in 1976 as the Best Hospital External Relations Program for Overall Community Service in the MacEachern Award competition.

1970 HORSE INVADES HOSPITAL? Friends, intending to visit a 15-year-old Peralta patient, smuggle a horse into the medical facility. They

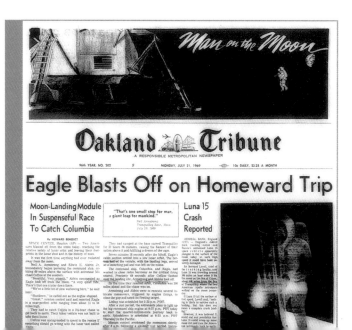

Man meets moon, Oakland Tribune, July, 1969

make it into the elevator, but are prevented from reaching the patient's bedside.

1971 Taking on a new name as the Golden State Warriors, the National Basketball Association team moves across the Bay to Oakland and holds court at the new Oakland-Alameda County Coliseum Arena.

1971 Peralta adds fluorescent angiography equipment (purchased for $32,000), a new argon laser photoagulator, and the East Bay's first linear accelerator for cancer treatment.

1971 The East Bay Health Foundation recommends consolidation of services by four hospitals: Merritt, Peralta, Providence, and Children's. All four boards agree in principle. The recommendation is based on a study by SRI, formerly Stanford Research Institute. This same year, Merritt, Peralta, Providence, and Children's hospitals establish a shared services corporation called Administrative Hospital Services Inc.

1971 Herrick introduces the East Bay's first methadone maintenance treatment program to rehabilitate heroin addicts.

Other developments: Bylaws of Herrick's Board of Trustees and Medical Staff are revised. The Board of Trustees increases to 12 members elected at-large, with the presidents of the Medical Staff and Herrick Memorial Hospital Guild also serving.

1972 Merritt demolishes its old South Wing, the last of its original buildings. A new building is planned for the site, which will include 30 beds, radiology, surgery, a Coronary Care Unit, special services for joint replacement, and a Microsurgical Unit.

1972 BART, headquartered in Oakland, begins operations. (Construction had begun in 1964.)

1972 Alta Bates establishes new departments of gastroenterology and nephrology, a new Respiratory Care Unit and a new parking structure debut.

1972 PROVIDENCE CLOSES ITS NURSING COLLEGE. With enrollment dwindling, the Sisters decide to close the College of Nursing after 68 years and graduating 1,515 nurses.

1972 The Babington Regional Kidney Center, a chronic renal dialysis facility, introduces care for patients who live in Alameda, Contra Costa, Napa, and Solano counties. The center is named in honor of the late Suren H. Babington, MD, former president of Herrick's Board of Trustees and founder, in 1947, of the hospital's medical teaching programs for interns and residents.

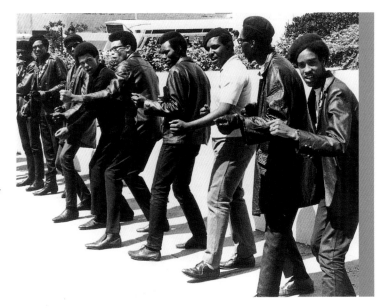

Supporters at the 1968 trial of Huey P. Newton, who co-founded the Black Panther Party in Oakland in 1966 Opposite: Susanne Jackson, RN, longtime Alta Bates employee, visits with a patient, 1970.

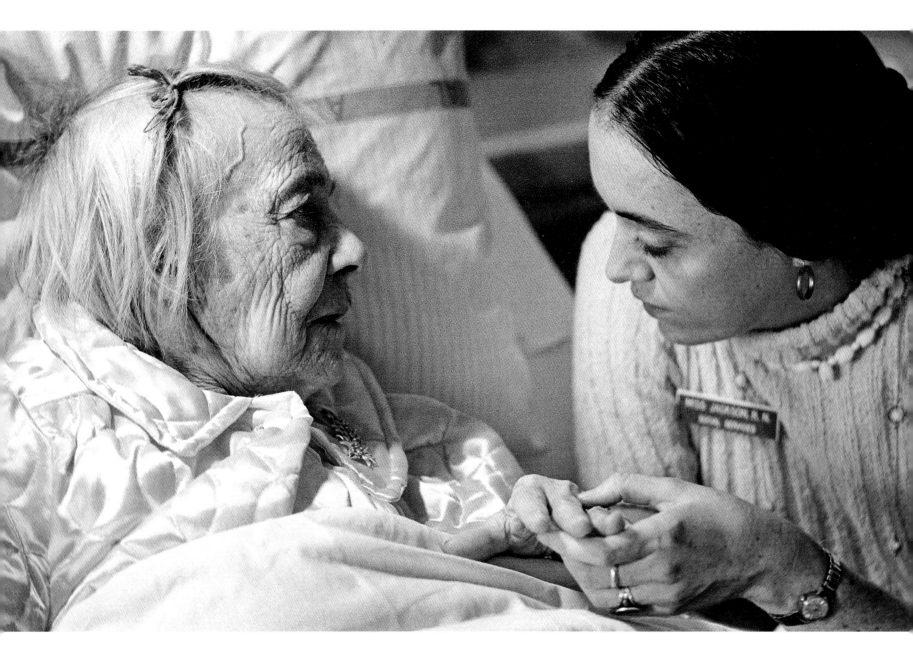

"Today's hospital cares for the sick, but must do more. It must carry on functions through which a modern hospital serves its community: patient care, public health, research, and education."

—Alfred Maffly, Herrick Hospital administrator

When the Department of Radiology is remodeled and expanded, Herrick becomes the first East Bay hospital to have a remote-controlled fluoroscope and an X-ray machine designed exclusively for mammography.

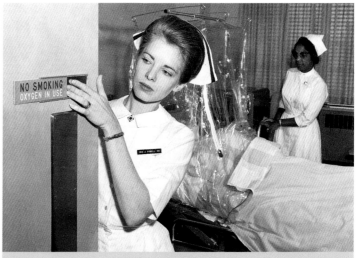

A Peralta nurse clears the air—and safeguards patients.

1972 Alta Bates extends its emergency care to 24-hour service.

1973 PROVIDENCE DIVERSIFIES. Providence opens its Pastoral Care Department to serve the spiritual needs of the sick. The staff is composed of highly qualified religious personnel of various denominations who combine up-to-date counseling techniques with the traditional work of the sisters in their compassionate visits to the sick and dying.

In response to the sophistication of modern medicine, a Medical Morals Committee outlines a code of ethics for patient treatment. Also this year and the next, Coagulation, Vestibular, Endocrine-Metabolic, and Gastroenterology laboratories are established. An Ostomy Care Program will begin in 1976. The following year, Providence is designated as the base emergency care facility for North Oakland, the downtown area, Emeryville, and Piedmont.

1973 Members of the radical Symbionese Liberation Army slay Marcus Foster, the first African American schools superintendent in Oakland.

1973 Computerized axial tomography (CAT) is invented by Sir Godfrey Newbold Hounsfield and Allan Cormack in England and the United States, respectively.

1973 Using the hospital's newly installed, $16,000 operating microscope for replantation of limbs and digits, Merritt surgeon Jack Tupper, MD, performs the East Bay's first successful reattachment of an amputated finger. This same year, Dr. Jackson performs the East Bay's first knee replacement at Merritt, and same-day surgery debuts.

1973 Alta Bates develops several programs to provide needed services in a less costly manner. The Home Health Care Program provides nursing, physical therapy, and other medical services in the patient's home following hospitalization at Alta Bates. An Outpatient Department enables physicians to provide treatment in a hospital setting without the patient having to bear the cost of an overnight stay. Alta Bates also institutes a part-pay program for 200 obstetrical patients each year.

1973 Herrick's Disabled Community Health Clinic—the first of its kind in the nation—offers health maintenance care to the community's thousands of physically disabled people.

As part of its rehabilitation program, Herrick becomes the first community general hospital in the Bay Area to establish a unit specifically for

facts and figures

1974
MERRITT HOSPITAL

Patients hospitalized	12,749
Operations performed	6,867
Average length of stay	7.4 days
65 years and over	9.4 days
Under age 65	6.6 days
Emergency patients	8,784
% Medicare patients	34.2
Babies born	886
Lab tests	647,434

Kathryn Parsons and Ken Richmond explore the Hall of Health, 1974.

heart sounds

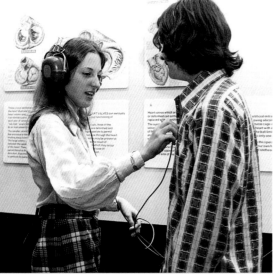

neurological patients who need continuous observation and treatment. Herrick also becomes the East Bay's first hospital to employ echocardiography (the use of ultrasound) to detect coronary abnormalities and disease.

1973 Peralta completes the first phase of its radiology remodeling project. Mammography services are introduced.

1973 The California State Department of Health inspects Providence and declares it does not meet seismic resistant criteria established by federal legislative action. (A 1974 earthquake study will show that the Hayward Fault lies in direct proximity to the hospital.) Providence, along with many other institutions in the Bay Area, will have to be redesigned in accordance with seismic resistant standards. Plans for a new hospital are begun immediately.

1974 The Oakland A's are victors in the World Series (their third in a row) over the Los Angeles Dodgers.

1974 Alta Bates receives the highest score of the 17 hospitals selected by the U.S. Department of Health, Education and Welfare to participate in a Nursing Quality Care Study. In this same year, the hospital's nationally acclaimed hands-on health education program, the Hall of Health, opens its doors to the public.

1974 Herrick and Alta Bates hospitals jointly receive a $50,000 federal grant to explore the feasibility of establishing an HMO (Health Maintenance Organization). The in-depth study project is dubbed HEALS—for <u>Herrick</u>-<u>Al</u>ta Bates <u>S</u>tudy.

1975 A NEW PROVIDENCE GETS UNDER WAY. Hundreds of guests attend groundbreaking ceremonies for the construction of a new Providence on the site where the School of Nursing once stood. The third hospital of the

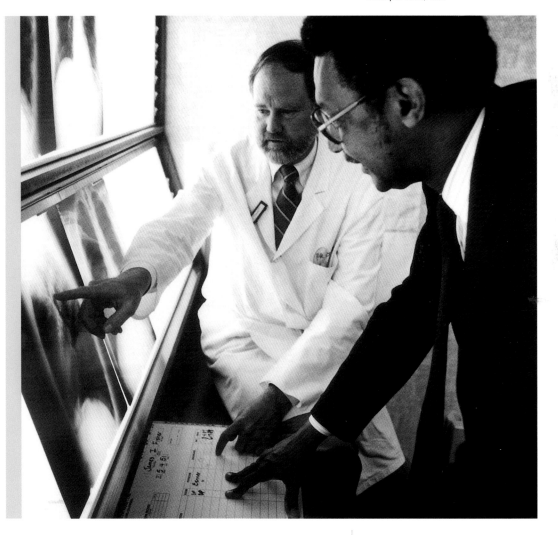

A medical consultation at Merritt between Less Chafen, MD, and Joseph Clift, MD

Sisters of Providence in Oakland, this multistoried structure of approximately 200,000 square feet will consist of a four-story nursing tower and an additional wing for special-care inpatients. Four

(continued on page 76)

babies, babies, babies

In 1964, Alta Bates names its new nursery after Hubert Long, MD, the longtime Berkeley pediatrician who may have administered more childhood immunizations—and comforted more new moms—than any physician in the area. Dr. Long succinctly states his philosophy of "new individuals," his pet name for newborns: "They're rugged little people," he tells the *Berkeley Daily Gazette*, "who thrive on anything."

Love for all the "little people" and absolute dedication to their care has been a proud tradition and will remain a standard of excellence at Alta Bates Summit Medical Center in 2004. Hundreds of thousands of babies have been born at Alta Bates, Herrick, Merritt, Providence, and Peralta over the last 100 years. Chances are good, if you were born in a Berkeley or Oakland hospital, the first view you saw in this world—after your mother's adoring smile, of course—was one of our nurseries.

Maternity services and the birthing experience have changed with the times. Deliveries at East Bay hospitals increase dramatically, for example, after World War II. Here and across the nation, maternity wards witness the advent of the famous Baby Boom. In 1935, just 37 percent of births nationwide occurred in hospitals; by 1949, driven by concerns over infant mortality rates, that figure had jumped to 87 percent.

More cases in point: Alta Bates rose from 635 births in 1940 to 1,865 in 1950. In 1938, Merritt Hospital delivered 872 babies; ten years later, that number spiked to 2,242. Interestingly, the Baby Boom declines in the mid-'50s in Oakland and other urban centers, as the population shifts to the suburbs.

The '60s and '70s witness renewed interest in home births among women who dislike institutional settings. Hospitals will respond in the '80s with labor and delivery rooms featuring the comforts of home and will allow women to choose their birth experience and invite participants. (No more Fathers' Waiting Rooms!)

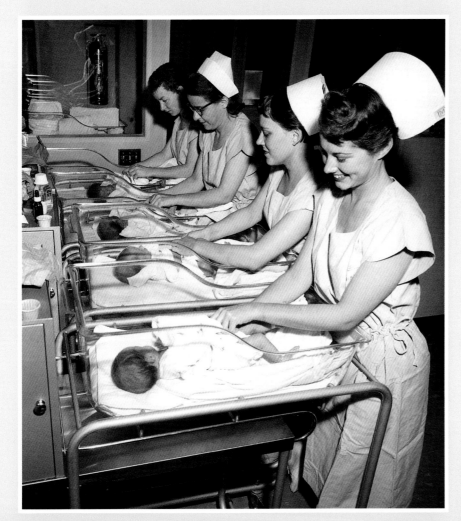

The Hoskins quadruplets in 1958, proud progeny of a Merritt physician

By 2004, more than 10,000 babies will be born annually at Alta Bates Summit. Each birth will enjoy services and facilities that far exceed capabilities of maternity wards just a few decades ago. In 1998, Alta Bates will complete a $7 million redesign of the Newborn Intensive Care Unit (NICU). The refurbished NICU will combine family-friendly services with state-of-the-art technology—all administered with loving care and provided in a soothing environment—the first of its kind in the nation.

Happily, most of the thousands of deliveries over the years were routine procedures, but the hospitals have also witnessed their share of extraordinary births—some that made local, even national, headlines. Here are a few notables:

• Alta Bates made local medical history in 1932 when three sets of twins were born here on October 16.

• In 1958, Dr. and Mrs. Dean Hoskins (a physician on the Merritt Hospital medical staff) become the proud parents of quadruplets, three girls and a boy, delivered at Merritt Hospital.

• Twenty years later, three sets of triplets are born at Merritt in a 10-week period—a three-in-one-million chance occurrence. "Expressing this small probability in a different way," quips Cal statistician Gordon Weiss, PhD, "three triplet births at Merritt within 10 weeks can be expected again in about 60,000 years."

• In 1984, six years after the first test-tube baby was born in England, Alta Bates will establish its renowned In Vitro Fertilization Program. In 1986, the hospital's first test-tube babies will be born.

• By 2004, more than 25,000 newborns will be listed on Alta Bates' Cradle Roll, a special program that's raised thousands of dollars each year since its inception in the '50s. Over the decades, relatives of these honored babies have generously donated to the hospital and proudly strolled the hallways of Alta Bates to view endearing displays of the children's names.

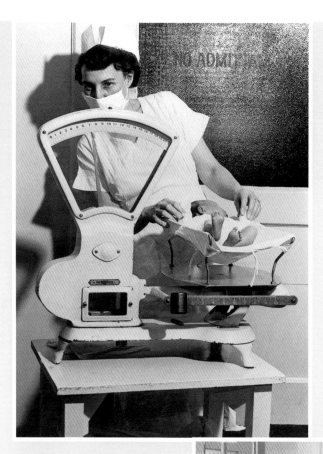

Left: Weight watching at Alta Bates, circa 1955
Below: Birth at Providence, circa 1950s

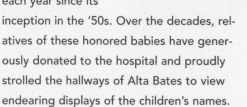

years and $22.5 million later, the completed 230-bed hospital will be ready for dedication.

1975 Herrick's Department of Nuclear Medicine is established. The laboratory is modernized and a total body scanning system added.

1975 ALTA BATES DEDICATES NEW WING. Inclement weather aside, some 2,000 people arrive on October 26 to help dedicate Alta Bates new $17 million wing.

All the beds in the 1928 building are replaced and total bed capacity reaches 311. The two north towers house Admitting; the Business Office; Social Services; Discharge Planning; administrative and nursing offices; Medical Records; Personnel; a cafeteria; an auditorium; the Education and Training Center; classroom and conference rooms; a doctor's lounge and library; a quiet room;

Alta Bates surgery suite, 1975

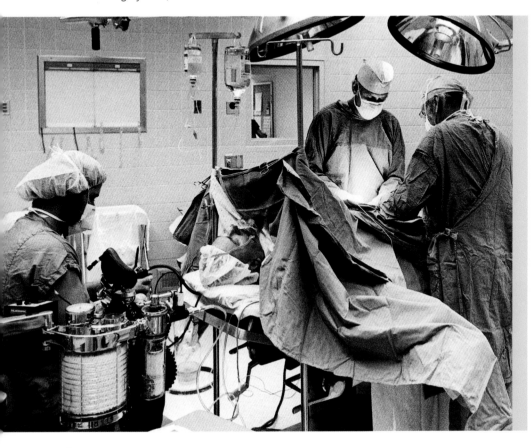

Housekeeping; Materials Management; and the office of the Alta Bates Volunteer Association.

The hospital now has a new Maternity-Infant Care Center, new areas for patient and community education, and expanded diagnosis and support services. A new Gift Shop opens on the first floor and, in 1976, a portion of the main lobby becomes the Alta Bates Art Gallery. In 1977, the Outpatient Department moves into its own area, separate from Emergency; and Surgery Day Care, the Vascular Laboratory, and the Alternative Birth Center open.

Beyond the physical growth of this period, the hospital dramatically expands its scope of services, creating about 15 different specialty centers under contract with physicians. This innovative arrangement will transform the facility from local hospital to leading medical center.

1975 Alta Bates Foundation incorporates as a separate organization. The Alta Bates Foundation Associates is established as a community volunteer group to help raise funds. The group opens a successful thrift shop, the Alta Bates Showcase.

1976 Peralta furthers its commitment to cancer care and research in establishing its Oncology Unit. The Peralta Research Institute, a joint effort between the University of California and Peralta, opens.

1976 The first Apple computer hits the market.

1976 Merritt, Peralta, and Providence cooperate to establish the first CT scanner on Pill Hill.

1977 HERRICK KICKS OFF PROJECT 80. Phase I of Herrick's long-range physical development program begins with groundbreaking ceremonies at the construction site of a five-story, 153-bed patient care wing. This wing will replace obsolescent facilities and adjoins the existing North

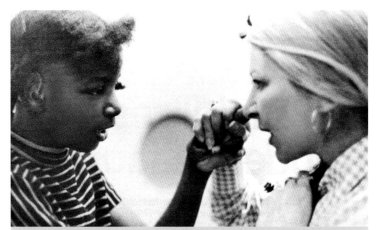

Herrick audiologist Linda Begen (later, Linda Peltz, a future hospital and Foundation board member) aids a deaf child's speech, 1976.

Also this year: Peralta opens its Chemical Dependency Hospital, installs a CAT scanner, and debuts use of the East Bay's only hyperbaric oxygen chamber (for use on cases such as smoke inhalation, skin grafts, and crush injuries).

1978 To enhance services for moms-to-be, Alta Bates introduces high-risk obstetrical care.

1978 Samuel Merritt Hospital Board of Directors approves Articles of Incorporation and bylaws of new Merritt Hospital Foundation.

1978–1979 Alta Bates and Herrick introduce Adult Sickle Cell Disease Programs. Alta Bates' program is conducted in close cooperation with several other major institutions, including the University of California, San Francisco General Hospital, and Children's Hospital.

1979 THE NEW PROVIDENCE IS DEDICATED. The new 230-bed Providence Hospital opens at the site of its old College of Nursing, just north of the 1926 building, at 3100 Summit Street. In conformance with all seismic requirements, this modern facility consists primarily of single-patient rooms with private baths and is fully air-conditioned and carpeted.

1979 The World Health Organization declares the eradication of smallpox.

1979 Alta Bates purchases and renovates Albany Hospital. The facility reopens in December as a rehabilitation and general acute care hospital.

Wing, matching it and the South Wing at each floor level. The construction cost is $9.8 million.

Also this year: Herrick acquires a $500,000 CAT scanner and introduces the Retinal Photography and Gastroenterology departments. The Alameda County Board of Supervisors designates Herrick as the primary emergency hospital for Zone 1 (Albany-Berkeley).

1977 PROVIDENCE IS 75. May 24 marks the 75th Anniversary of the official founding of Providence. Congratulations and proclamations come from the White House, California's Secretary of State, and the City of Oakland.

1977 A record Super Bowl crowd, joined by 81 million TV viewers, watches the Raiders win their first NFL championship.

1978 The first test-tube baby is born.

1978 PERALTA IS 50. On July 7, the hospital celebrates its 50th anniversary with the dedication of the Sherrick Building on Summit Street. Four months earlier, a dramatic phase of the Trustees' long-range development plan began with the construction of a three-level, 43,000-square-foot Outpatient Services Building.

Golden State Warriors' Phil Smith gets in SHAPE, the Peralta sports medicine program that debuts in 1979.

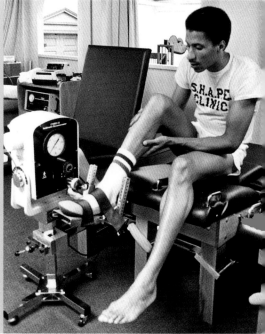

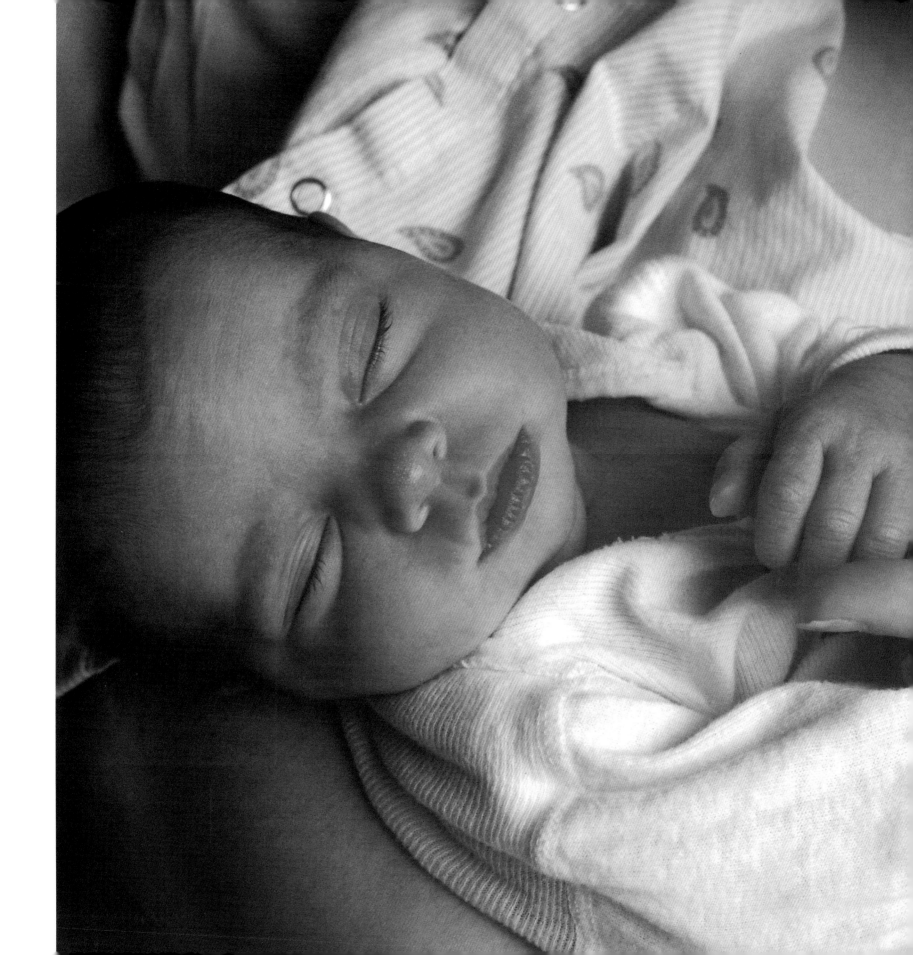

# of rebirth and renewal

Just three hours old. Welcome!

The 1980s, 1990s, and early 2000s are a period of adaptation and consolidation for Alta Bates, Herrick, Merritt, Peralta, and Providence hospitals. More than any other factor, economics drives institutional change as these health care facilities face high demand for their services and revenue shortfalls brought on, in part, by Medicare and Medi-Cal obligations.

In 1982, Merritt and Peralta merge; in 1988, Alta Bates and Herrick officially follow suit. Merritt Peralta and Providence create a single Pill Hill entity in 1992, Summit Medical Center. All join in 1999 to constitute the 1,000-bed Alta Bates Summit Medical Center. In the chronology of these consolidations, common goals can be readily identified—namely, provision of quality health care, efficient allocation of resources, and prompt response to patient needs and community emergencies (such as the 1989 Loma Prieta earthquake and the 1991 firestorm).

Across decades that witness the fall of the Soviet Union, the rise of personal computing, the emergence of AIDS, the impeachment of a U.S. president, the bursting of the dotcom bubble (and the return of the Raiders), the hospitals set their landmarks. Merritt pioneers balloon angioplasty in the East Bay; Alta Bates establishes Northern California's first community hospital–based Bone Marrow Transplantation Program; and Alta Bates Summit introduces surgical robotics in Oakland and Berkeley. With renewed commitment, a stronger-than-ever medical center accepts the challenge of its next 100 years—and beyond.

1980

1980s Berkeley emerges from the turmoil of the 1960s and 1970s with a few changes, including major shifts in culture, demographics, and politics. In fact, Berkeley's population actually declines about 12 percent in the 1970s and 1980s as the city enacts growth measures to improve quality over quantity.

In the 1980s and 1990s the University of California student body emphasizes academics rather than issues, and admission standards at Cal hit an unprecedented high.

1980s Oakland takes a slow but marked turn toward rebirth. Oakland's center at 14th and

1980–1989:
U.S. population: 226,546,000
Berkeley population (1980): 103,328
Oakland population (1980): 339,337
Life expectancy: male, 69.9; female, 77.6
Average salary: $15,757/year
Minimum wage: $3.10/hour
BMW cost: $12,000; Mercedes 280 E cost: $14,800
Movie attendance: 20 million/week
In 1989, Americans gave $115,000,000,000 to charity
Source: HandPrints, *Children's Hospital Oakland*

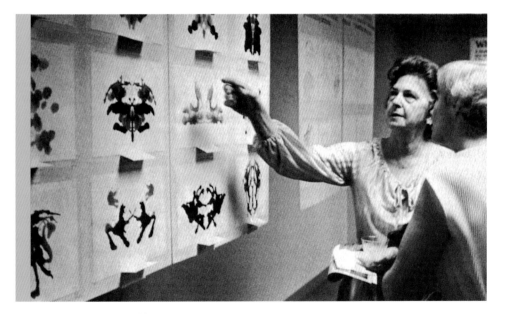

Intrigued by an inkblot display, guests tour new psychiatric facilities at Herrick Hospital, 1980.

the hospital continues to reach out to Oakland's community and provide for their needs. Steps are taken to serve those who are often forgotten, including the poor and the elderly. Proposals include programs for offering hot meals, food and clothing, and Adult Day Health Care—assistance sorely needed but expensive to implement.

Additional specialty programs are launched, such as the Metabolic Bone Institute for the treatment of osteoporosis and other bone diseases and the Diabetic and Endocrine Institute for the treatment of diabetes and related illness. These programs are unique in the Bay Area and offer the community local specialized services.

Broadway blossoms, and the grand City Center complex takes shape; the Port of Oakland once again takes its place as pacesetter and wins distinction as the nation's second largest container port.

1980s In looking toward its future and responding to Oakland's changes, Providence Hospital develops strategies for the '80s. To fulfill the Sisters' mission,

1980 HERRICK HOSPITAL DEDICATES NEW WING. Some 270 people brave the weather for the first ever Herrick Health Run, part of the festivities celebrating the hospital's new 153-bed wing. Many Herrick employees and members of the medical staff participate in the 2.5- and 4.7-mile run through Berkeley streets.

The new wing facilitates a doubling of emergency services and features a new surgical suite, state-of-the-art radiology equipment, and new environments for medical, surgical, psychiatric, and rehab patients.

1980 Samuel Merritt Hospital will need about $16 million over the next five years for capital equipment and program needs, according to a report to the Merritt Hospital Foundation board. This same year, General Foods provides a $25,000 grant for South Wing remodeling.

Other developments: Merritt kicks off a new employee shuttle service called Van Am BART (a play on the name of a popular local TV personality) and starts the Lifeline program to connect patients to emergency assistance, should they need it. The Kilpatrick Coronary Care Unit is named for a donor whose lifetime gifts total more than $450,000.

1980 ALTA BATES HOSPITAL IS 75. The hospital marks the occasion with gala festivities enjoyed by hundreds of community supporters, hospital administrators, and medical staff members. This same year, Alta Bates Volunteer Association celebrates 25 years and 1,000,000 hours of service.

1981 Samuel Merritt Hospital College of Nursing, in cooperation with Saint Mary's College of California in Moraga, offers the West's first four-year intercollegiate nursing program jointly sponsored by a hospital and a college and features a bachelor of science degree in nursing.

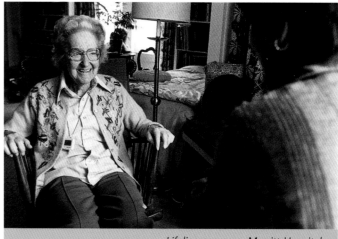

Lifeline program, Merritt Hospital

1981 IBM's personal computer hits the market.

1981 Peralta Medical Foundation is reactivated.

1981 Acquired immune deficiency syndrome (AIDS) is recognized as a new disease.

1981 The Alta Bates Corporation is formed. By 1986, this corporation will own and operate three acute-care hospitals and have a contract to manage a fourth. It also will own 17 skilled nursing facilities, four intermediate-care facilities, two residential/community-care facilities, and 13 housing/independent living centers, and provide home health care through two visiting nurses' associations and clinical laboratory services through its Pathology Institute subsidiary.

1981 As do other hospitals of the day, Alta Bates experiences escalating problems with Medicare and Medi-Cal reimbursements. An excerpt from Alta Bates' Annual Report: *"In 1981, Alta Bates Hospital did not receive*

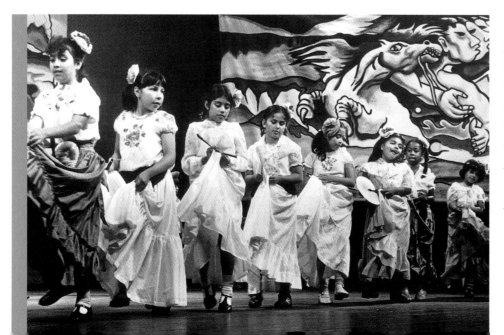

Celebrating Cinco de Mayo in Oakland, circa 1980s

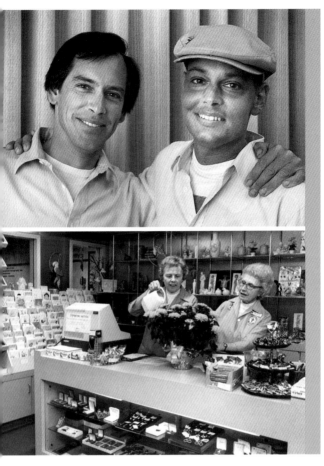

Top: John Werner (right), first patient in Alta Bates Hospital's bone marrow transplant program (headed by Jeffrey L. Wolf, MD) and his brother Patrick, who donated the marrow,1984
Bottom: Providence Hospital Gift Shop volunteers Eva Curotto (left) and Louise Sullivan, 1982

$14,276,000, the difference between our charges and what the government reimbursed for Medicare and Medi-Cal services. This sum is more than double what it cost Alta Bates in 1980 ($7,042,000), and more than seven times our excess revenue over expense...."*

Excerpts from a patient letter to the hospital (published in a 1982 issue of *Alta Bates News*):

"... I am shocked to learn that the cost to the hospital of all the fine care given me is not fully covered by Medicare. In this there seems some degree of injustice; but more practically, I can see that your fine hospital cannot indefinitely continue its high-quality service to its patients under such economics."

1982 MERRITT PIONEERS IN ANGIOPLASTY.

Continuing its tradition as a premier center for heart care, Merritt is the first hospital in the East Bay to apply the breakthrough cardiovascular technique of balloon angioplasty in treatment of blocked coronary arteries.

1982 MERRITT AND PERALTA MERGE.

Effective in January, Peralta and Merritt merge to form Merritt Peralta Medical Center (MPMC). This marks the first time in the East Bay that two independent hospitals have consolidated.

They form a not-for-profit parent corporation and together comprise the largest heath care facility in the East Bay. With a total of 630 beds,

they serve over 20,000 inpatients and nearly 150,000 outpatients annually.

This same year, Zella Daniels, RN, leaves $103,000 to Peralta for medical research. The Peralta Cancer Research Institute becomes an independent institution. Sean R. Althaus, MD, performs Merritt's first cochlear implant. The hospital is one of 22 national centers that are experimenting with the procedure.

1982 An artificial heart is implanted into a human in the United States by Willem Kolff, MD, PhD, keeping the patient alive for 112 hours. Insulin becomes the first genetically engineered hormone to be approved by the U. S. Food and Drug Administration (FDA).

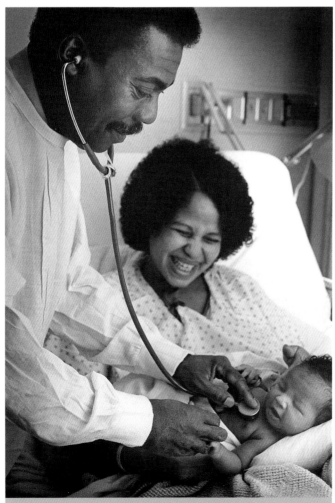

Robert Minera, MD, checks an Alta Bates newborn, 1981.

1982 The California Assembly passes three health care bills, and the federal government creates the Tax and Equity Fiscal Responsibility Act (TEFRA). This legislation drastically changes the way hospitals are reimbursed for their services, spawning a decade of change, downsizing, and competition.

1983 **ALTA BATES INTRODUCES BONE MARROW TRANSPLANTATION.** In conjunction with Children's Hospital Oakland, Alta Bates begins the Bone Marrow Transplantation Program, the first community hospital–based program of its kind in Northern California.

1983 Rich McCann, CEO and president of MPMC, reports an estimated $8 million will be needed for Merritt's fifth-floor renovation and from $3 million to $27 million for demolition and replacement of the Peralta Tower. McCann says about $40 million will be needed for construction and $10 million for equipment in the next decade.

1983 **NEW LEADERSHIP COMES TO PROVIDENCE HOSPITAL.** Late this year, Sister Dona Taylor is named Administrator of Providence. Momentum picks up quickly as new programs and services get underway. Lithotripsy, home and occupational health care, and specialized cancer care programs are implemented.

1984 The first surgery is performed on a fetus in utero. The FDA approves magnetic resonance imaging (MRI).

1984 Alta Bates and Herrick affiliate. Acute Care Affiliates is established as a hospital holding company under the auspices of the Alta Bates Corporation.

Under the medical direction of Richard Chetkowski, MD, Alta Bates introduces its In Vitro

building a tradition

1980–1998

ALTA BATES HERRICK

1980 New 153-bed wing at Herrick
1983 Alta Bates' 1928 building demolished
1985 New three-story structure dedicated at Alta Bates; replaces the 1928 building
1998 Debut of $7 million, 55-bed Newborn Intensive Care Unit at Alta Bates

MERRITT PERALTA

1985 The Merritt Peralta Health Education Center opens; $3 million renovation of Merritt's maternity department and nursery begins.
1986 5 South, an innovative model nursing wing, opens.

PROVIDENCE

1988 Dedication of $3 million, 61,000–square-foot Providence Medical Office building
1991 24-bed Skilled Nursing Facility opens.

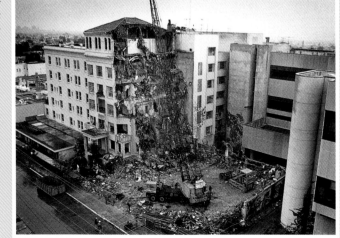

Demolition of Alta Bates' 1928 building

Fertilization program. *American Health* magazine (October 1989) will later report that the program has earned a reputation as one of the "top 10 infertility clinics in the country."

1985 Thanks to thousands of generous donors, the Merritt Peralta Health Education Center opens to the community. The medical center begins a $3 million renovation of its maternity department and nursery.

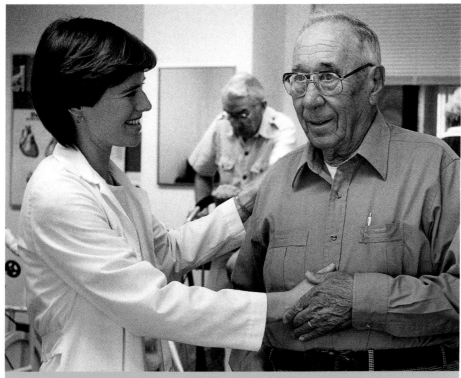

In good hands with Herrick's Rehabilitation Services, circa 1980s

Other developments: Merritt Peralta merges with Delta Memorial Hospital, a 53-bed community hospital in Antioch. The new MRI technology is employed in a facility below the Peralta site.

1985 Alameda Hospital signs a management contract with Alta Bates Corporation, and Alta Breast Center opens at 5730 Telegraph Avenue. Its streamlined service includes BSE (breast self-examination) training as well as dedicated breast health specialists. The state-of-the-art MRI facility allows women to receive mammograms free of radiation. In its first year, 3,000 women receive checkups, and 30 cases are detected.

1985 A twin-engine plane slams into the Sun Valley Mall just two days before Christmas, killing four and injuring at least 75. Nine victims of the fiery crash are treated at the Alta Bates Burn Center.

1985 Merritt Peralta initiates the Home Calls program of visiting nurses and health aides.

1985 The Northern California Alzheimer's Disease Center opens at Herrick.

1986 MERRITT OPENS MODEL NURSING WING. Merritt opens 5 South, an innovative model nursing wing. At the reception celebrating the opening, a Merritt Peralta Foundation donor provides a major gift to sponsor the Elizabeth Hinds Jamieson Suite in the remodeled general nursing unit.

Also this year: The 10,000th cardiac catheterization is performed at the Cardiac Catheterization Laboratory, and the Community Health Advisory Board begins meeting. A sign of the financial times: There are eight patients at Merritt in February whose care has cost $1,880,000, while the Medicare reimbursement provides only $123,000. The Merritt Peralta Foundation transfers $300,000 to provide for the care of heart patients in this group.

1986 A tiny television is added to the modern laparoscope, making a major advance in "keyhole" surgery.

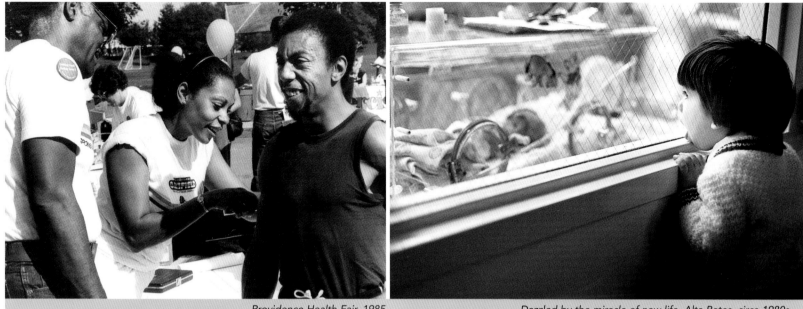

Providence Health Fair, 1985

Dazzled by the miracle of new life, Alta Bates, circa 1980s

1986 OB IS REBORN AT PROVIDENCE.
Providence opens its Family Birthing Unit, after a lapse of over 10 years of obstetrical services. The unit features private rooms, single-bed birthing, and a family-centered concept. Alta Bates' Alternative Birth Center, which shares this innovative approach, debuted in 1977.

1986 It is estimated that the average patient at Alta Bates and Herrick uses 18.9 pounds of laundry a day. Alta Bates' switchboard handles 5,000 calls daily. More than 8,000 surgeries are performed a year at the two hospitals: inpatient 5,200; outpatient 2,900. Also, in 1986, 430 volunteers donate a record 79,495 hours of service.

1987 Merritt's Cancer Education and Prevention program opens, based on a prior breast-screening project at the hospital. Also this year, Merritt's board of directors approves the transfer of selected assets to the newly independent Board of Regents of Samuel Merritt College of Nursing.

1987 ADULT DAY HEALTH CARE DEBUTS AT PROVIDENCE. The hospital is the first in the Oakland community to offer such a program.

1987 Alta Bates introduces the East Bay AIDS Center, the first of its kind in the nation. This same year, Peralta opens an Adult Immunology clinic to

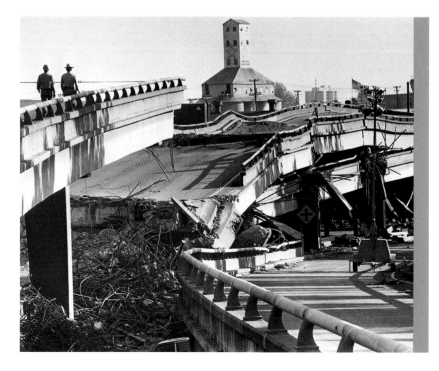

East Bay hospitals and emergency services rally to the rescue when the 1989 earthquake collapses portions of the Cypress interchange.

care for patients who have HIV/AIDS and installs a lithotripter.

1987 Prozac is introduced.

1987–1988 Although affiliated, Alta Bates and Herrick continue to operate as freestanding hospitals through 1987. Each has its own administrative and medical staffs and operates separate emergency departments, medical-surgical programs, and intensive care units. Responding to an ever more challenging operating environment, the hospitals merge on January 1, 1988, and the organization is renamed Alta Bates Herrick Hospital. They become a single legal entity, with one medical staff, operating on two complementary hospital sites. Duplication of services ends; medical/surgical and emergency services are consolidated at the Alta Bates site.

It becomes more and more clear that stand-alone hospitals are not going to survive. In an effort to further develop an East Bay and San Francisco delivery system, Alta Bates Corporation and Children's Hospital in San Francisco agree to affiliate.

1988 New technologies boost the cell phone industry. (The first working prototype was demonstrated in 1973.)

1988 PROVIDENCE DEDICATES $13.5 MILLION MEDICAL OFFICE BUILDING. During Sister Dona's last year as Providence Hospital administrator, she facilitates dedication of one of the decade's largest projects. The 61,000–square-foot Providence Medical Office Building is located at the site of the 1926 hospital. The stunning structure includes physician office suites, an in-house

Merritt Peralta Institute (MPI) is the Bay Area's first hospital-based treatment program for substance abuse. By 2003—MPI's 25th anniversary—more than 15,000 individuals will find help there.

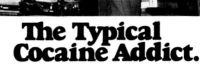

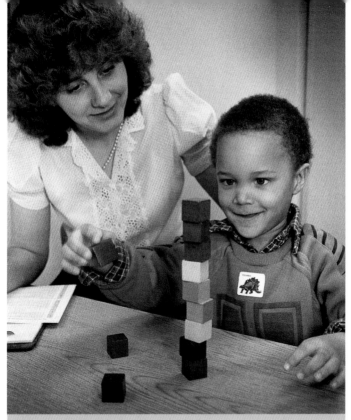

In Herrick's Small Voice program, Ahmeer Lewis builds communication skills, aided by speech pathologist Carolyn Rose, 1987.

pharmacy, laboratory, radiology, and food services and features a two-story atrium lobby, glassed walls throughout, and skyline views.

1988 A vascular laser is employed at Merritt Peralta to open blocked leg arteries. This equipment is furnished partly through the generosity of the Hedco Foundation and other donors to the Merritt Peralta Foundation. This year, the Foundation holds a successful celebrity fundraiser starring Dionne Warwick and Burt Bacharach. Over $85,000 is raised for the maternity and nursery renovation.

1988 The Peralta Eye Center opens.

1989 EARTHQUAKE STRIKES. On October 17 at 5:04 p.m., a 7.1 earthquake shakes the Loma Prieta fault in the Santa Cruz Mountains, causing $5.9 billion in property damage and 63 deaths. Buildings collapse in San Francisco's Marina District and a section of the Bay Bridge collapses, as do portions of the Cypress interchange connecting Freeway 880 with the Bay Bridge. In Oakland, the temblor displaces more than 2,500 people, damages 200 businesses and 1,400 homes, and injures 320 people. The World Series is delayed by the quake but concludes with an Oakland A's win over the San Francisco Giants.

1989 Alta Bates Herrick, Providence, and Merritt Peralta implement their emergency triage systems and treat earthquake victims from around the Bay Area. The Pill Hill hospitals operate under emergency power.

1989 On New Year's Eve, Tim and Maria Lasignan become parents of quadruplets, the first to be born at Alta Bates Herrick.

1990 The World Wide Web is first deployed as a working system.

1990 Chang-Lin Tien is appointed chancellor of the University of California at Berkeley and becomes the first Asian American to head a major U.S. university.

1990 Alta Bates Corporation (ABC) divests portions of its holdings, including American River Hospital and Eskaton (a Northern California provider of health, housing, and social services for seniors), because it was not feasible to build a health care delivery system for all of California. Instead, ABC focuses on developing a delivery system for the East Bay and San Francisco areas.

Left: Staff at a Disabled Community Health Clinic planning meeting, circa 1980s (left to right)—Mickey Scornaienchi, Barbara Baumann, MD, and Ann Cupolo
Center: Merritt linear accelerator
Right: Peralta lab

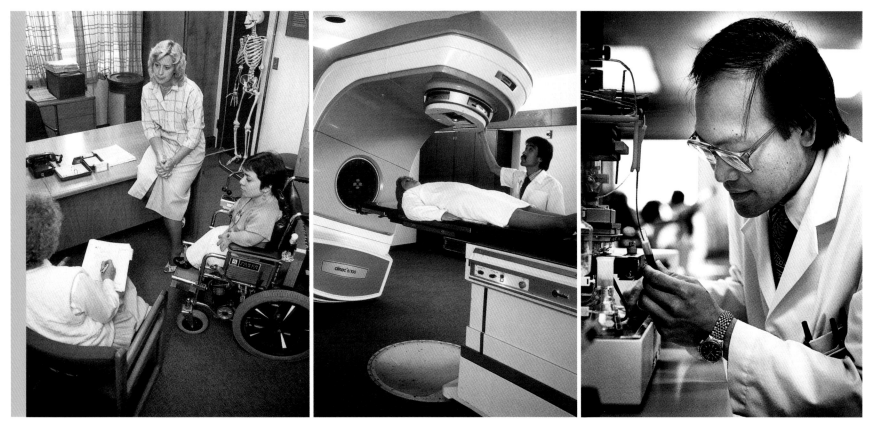

1990 Alta Bates Herrick's Adult Sickle Cell Program has achieved national recognition as a model treatment and education program for individuals with this chronic disease. This year, they receive a new Chevrolet van, courtesy of Oakland A's baseball star Ricky Henderson. Actor Danny Glover designates the program as recipient of $13,000 raised by KRON-TV through a benefit film premiere of *The Port Chicago Mutiny*.

1990 The Nutrition Labeling and Education Act requires all packaged foods to bear detailed nutrition labeling, including listing of color additives by name.

1991 The Soviet Union collapses.

1991 Thousands of reservists are called to the front lines in the Persian Gulf War, and many health professionals in the reserves step in to fill the now vacant slots in the Veteran's Administration system. Many of the reservists are children and grandchildren of Providence employees, medical staff, and auxiliaries. Providence holds Prayer for Peace services in its chapel and displays pictures of relatives or friends serving in the Mid-East as a show of support. The Persian Gulf War will end 40 days after it began.

1991 Health care delivery continues to change and adapt in response to more restrictive reimbursement policies. In

February, Providence opens a 24-bed Skilled Nursing Facility (SNF) for patients who no longer require acute care but are not ready for comprehensive rehabilitation, long-term convalescence in another facility, or recuperation at home.

1991 FIRESTORM RAGES. On October 20, Santa Ana winds and an out-of-control fire near the Caldecott Tunnel whip through the Oakland and Berkeley Hills. The inferno rages for 69 hours and burns 1,600 acres, leaving a staggering human toll of 25 dead, 150 injured, and 5,000 homeless.

1991 ALTA BATES AIDS FIRE VICTIMS. During the fire, Alta Bates is the closest hospital to assist fire victims, but is also on alert to evacuate its staff and patients. The Alta Bates Burn Center (soon to be named the DeNicolai Burn Center, after its generous benefactor) is absolutely critical during the firestorm, and afterward will receive a personal visit and commendation from Dr. Louis B. Sullivan, secretary of the U.S. Department of Health and Human Services. President George Bush also applauds the center and in a congratulatory letter writes, "The administrators, physicians, and nurses who came to the aid of their community at a time when their own homes were in jeopardy are true heroes." Alta Bates' Burn Center will be the first in the nation to use the new artificial skin transplant product, Integra, hailed as a breakthrough for burn patients.

The greater area health care community is hit particularly hard by the fire, since many physicians, employees, and volunteers live in the fire zone. According to a KCBS-AM radio report, 30 Alta Bates Herrick employees lose their residences. The blaze claims the life of one nurse, Kimberly Robson Dakis, RN, of the Alta Bates Medical Group.

Retired longshoreman Joseph Charles—known affectionately as The Waving Man—greets passing motorists in Berkeley, wearing his signature bright orange gloves. Charles happily manned his post for some 30 years (into the '90s), and once estimated that he cheered 4,500 passersby daily.

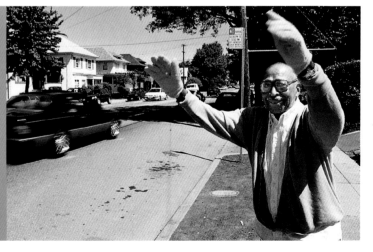

Opposite: The beating heart of a developing life delights both a mom-to-be and Alta Bates' OB/GYN Margaret Cuthbert, MD, 1986.

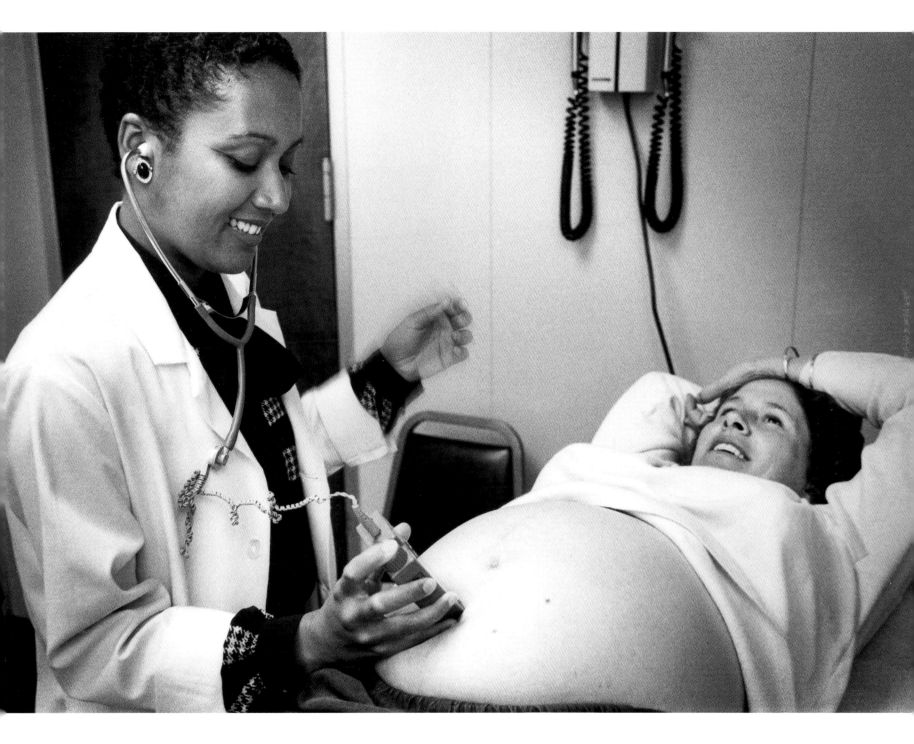

Our mission: We enhance the health and well-being of people in the communities we serve through compassion and excellence.

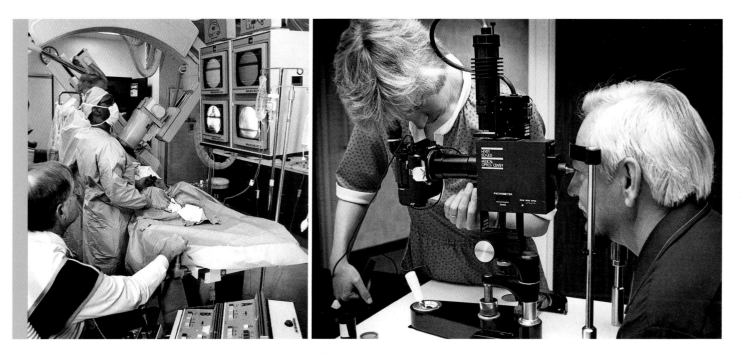

Left: Summit heart specialists introduce innovative techniques to East Bay cardiology, circa 1992–1993. Right: Seeing eye-to-eye at Peralta

Karen Bartolini, director of Providence's Adult Day Health Care, works with a program participant, circa 1990s.

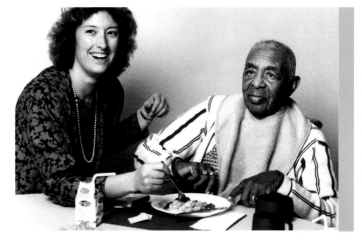

1991 PROVIDENCE PROVIDES FIRE RELIEF. Providence immediately responds to the firestorm as a Red Alert Zone 1 hospital. Physicians and hospital staff answer the call, many fulfilling their duties on-site, without knowing if their houses have survived the raging fire. The hospital treats 29 patients, most with "smoke inhalation" problems. Nine people are admitted, including Leo Pedemont, MD, a past president of the medical staff, and several fire fighters. Some 43 physicians, hospital staff, and auxiliary members lose or suffer severe damage to their homes from the fire. The hospital provides group counseling sessions and establishes a loan program for those affected.

1991 BERKELEY PRIMARY CARE ACCESS CLINIC OPENS AT HERRICK. The clinic provides community-based, subsidized services for uninsured and low-income residents of Berkeley, including obstetrical care, health education, postpartum care, family planning, and classes in parenting, pregnancy, and delivery. In 1995, the rent-free facility will undergo a $400,000 expansion, doubling in size.

1992 Alta Bates is recognized as the best hospital for care of mothers and babies, based on patient outcomes, in a report by the University of California and the California Department of Health Services. The hospital's new regional vascular center combines the expertise of vascular surgeons and interventional radiologists. Alta Bates is the first East Bay hospital to make use of a newly FDA-approved vascular stent in the treatment of vascular disease.

1992 ALTA BATES MEDICAL CENTER DEBUTS. In January, Alta Bates Herrick is renamed Alta Bates Medical Center.

1992 SUMMIT MEDICAL CENTER DEBUTS. On March 1, Providence and Merritt Peralta combine to establish Summit Medical Center.

The formation of a single, new health care organization promises better use of existing resources, elimination of many duplicative services, and expansion of others. A single entity with more resources also brings an improved ability to attract and retain top physicians, nurses, and other staff, and to implement new technologies.

Summit Medical Center's name is selected to reflect quality health care and excellence and to signify its hilltop location, a nod to the area's "Pill Hill" nickname. According to a U. S. Marketing Services report, other top picks were: New Metropolitan, Unity, Trinity, and East Bay Regional.

1992 Summit's Paul Ludmer, MD, and Michael Lee, MD, use radio frequency ablation to correct abnormal heart rhythms.

1992 KIDNAPPED NEWBORN IS RETURNED. Excerpts from *Hospital Security and Safety Management* (March 1993):

"The widely publicized Baby Kerri abduction, the first kidnapping in the 85-year-old history of Alta Bates, involved a two-day-old baby who was taken in June 1992 from a bassinet by a woman allegedly posing as a representative of a federally funded nutritional program for women, infants, and children. The baby was eventually reunited with her mother at the medical center last September after an intensive public awareness campaign and search effort by the medical center led to the arrest of the alleged kidnapper."

1992–1993 The Order of the Knights of Malta, a dedicated group of donors and volunteers at the new Summit Medical Center (and earlier at Providence), provide free flu shots to the needy, as well as financial support for the Adult Day Health Care Center. The order also works to add a clinic for Alzheimer's patients.

— THEN AND NOW —

a sound foundation

In 2004, Alta Bates Summit Foundation achieves record-setting fundraising sums and rallies vital community support for the Medical Center. Undoubtedly, the Foundation has benefitted from the stellar performance of its predecessors—the Alta Bates, Herrick, Merritt, Peralta, Providence, Merritt Peralta, Alta Bates Herrick, and Summit foundations. Activities in 2004, sponsored or co-sponsored by the Foundation, include:

Celebrity Golf and Tennis Classic: Since its start in 1993, this venue has become the nation's No. 1 celebrity tennis tournament and, by 2004, it raises a cumulative $3 million. The golf tourney,

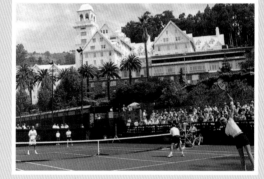

Annual celebrity tennis classic

which began as a Providence event in the '80s, is a perennial sellout.

Football 101: The site of this women-only fundraiser is the Oakland Raiders' headquarters. By 2004, the annual event (the brainchild of Summit enthusiasts) raises more than $100,000.

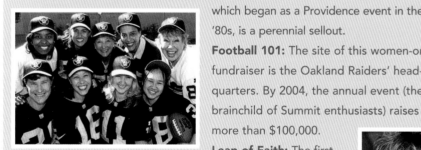

The team at Football 101

Leap of Faith: The first annual gala raises $100,000. It is co-hosted by Friends of Faith, a not-for-profit organization that seeks to improve access to breast cancer screening and services, and honors the memory of Faith Fancher, a local broadcast journalist and longtime breast cancer prevention advocate.

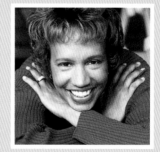

Honoring Faith Fancher

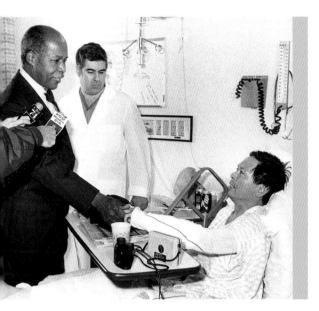

Dr. Louis B. Sullivan (left), secretary of the U.S. Department of Health and Human Services, tours the Alta Bates Burn Center with its medical director, Jerold Z. Kaplan, MD (center) and visits Berkeley optometrist Joseph Wong, a burn victim.

Summit Associates, formerly known as the Providence Century Club and the Merritt-Peralta Associates, is formed in 1993 to continue fundraising for the purchase of equipment, expansion of health care programs, and building renovations.

1993 Coyness Ennix, MD, and Summit surgeons perform their first coronary bypass without the use of a heart bypass machine. Summit Health Center opens at the Pacific Renaissance Health Center in Oakland's Chinatown.

1993 President Clinton signs The Family and Medical Leave Act.

1993 Oakland is designated an "All American City" by the National Civic League.

1993 The East Bay Medical Network is formed. Alta Bates Corporation changes its name to Alta Bates Health System. In 1994, Alta Bates affiliates with the California Healthcare System, a collaboration with some of the Bay Area's premier hospitals, including California Pacific Medical Center, Mills-Peninsula Hospitals, and Marin General Hospital.

1993 The first annual Alta Bates Celebrity Tennis Classic is held and nets an astounding $130,000.

1993 Led by Robert M. Greene, MD, Alta Bates' cardiac program is one of

the first in the nation to conduct research on clot-dissolving drugs under the TIMI IV (Thrombolysis in Myocardial Infarction) studies. Alta Bates is one of only four participating sites conducting this research in conjunction with Harvard Medical School.

1994 CNN lauds the Youth Bridge Mentoring Program as one of the best in the country. This program targets at-risk teens and teen parents and is a partnership between Alta Bates and the Berkeley Unified School District. Youth Bridge encourages young people to continue their education and to make successful transitions from adolescence to adulthood and the work place.

1995 Alta Bates' Breast Health Access for Women with Disabilities Clinic opens and is the first of its kind in the nation to provide comprehensive breast

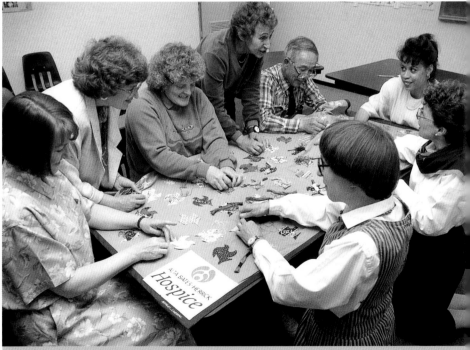

Crafting an AIDS quilt panel, Alta Bates Herrick Hospice and Visiting Nurse Association

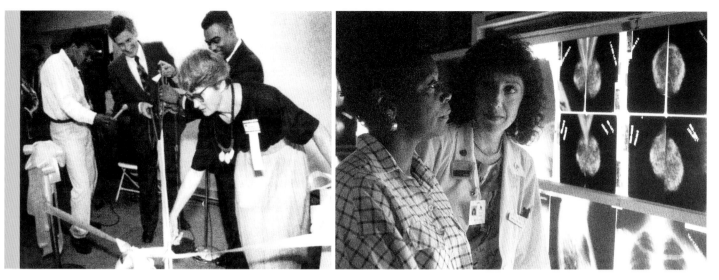

health services and educational outreach to women with serious motor impairments or disabilities. The clinic has a wheelchair-accessible mammography machine and special exam tables. Services are free to disabled women in Alameda and Contra Costa counties. The program will be instrumental in enhancing health care for disabled women nationwide.

1995 Summit is voted "Best Hospital" by the *Oakland Tribune* readers.

1995 After a 13-year "exile" in Los Angeles, the Raiders return to Oakland and their loyal fans. This same year, DVDs are introduced.

1996 SUMMIT DOCS INNOVATE. Summit cardiac surgeon Leigh Iverson, MD, introduces minimally invasive ("keyhole") procedures in bypass surgery. Summit physicians, including Dr. Ludmer, are the first in the nation to use a permanent pacemaker lead with a low pacing threshold to conserve energy. In 1997, Summit cardiologists are the first to deploy the Multilink stent, which in 2000 will become the most widely used device of its kind in the world.

1996 Sutter Health and California Healthcare System (CHS) affiliate.

1996 *Time* magazine names David Ho as its Man of the Year for his work in AIDS research. Ho's protease inhibitor "cocktail" treatment will add years to the lives of many AIDS patients.

1996 Summit's president and CEO, Irwin Hansen, wins the McEachern Award.

1997 The Alta Bates Foundation completes the largest and most successful capital campaign in its history, surpassing its $5 million goal by a laudable 40 percent.

1997 Summit's Ethnic Health Institute (EHI) is established to address the pressing health care needs of ethnic and underserved populations. A community service, EHI engages in health education, research, health provider training, and community outreach.

1997 In a historic collaboration, Kaiser Permanente's Oakland campus transfers its sizeable OB/GYN inpatient services to Alta Bates. The arrangement remains in effect until 2004.

Left: Norman Moscow, MD, president of the Alta Bates Herrick medical staff, assists Berkeley Mayor Loni Hancock in cutting the ribbon at the Berkeley Primary Care Access Clinic opening, 1991. Alameda County Supervisor Warren Widener (in dark suit) looks on.
Right: Reviewing mammograms at Summit Medical Center, 1993

1998 PSYCHIATRIC SERVICES RECORD 50-YEAR LANDMARK. Since 1948, Herrick has been a pioneering mental health provider in the East Bay. Its inpatient psychiatric services are a well-established and much relied on resource. Services include three levels of care for psychiatric inpatients: a closed unit for the most disorganized patients; an open unit for those making progress through counseling and individualized plans of care; and services for patients who require less intensive care and shorter periods of hospitalization.

In addition, the hospital has established a wide range of psychiatric services, including 24-hour emergency consultation service and clinical, referral, and information services on an outpatient basis. Herrick also introduced the first inpatient adolescent program in its service area.

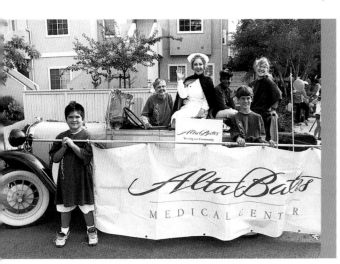

At Berkeley's first "How Berkeley Can You Be?" parade, September, 1996: (left to right) Nick Jones; Mary Baptista, driver/owner of the 1928 Model A Ford; Lisa Goines, RN, who portrayed hospital founder Alta Bates; Brittany Boyd; Zachary Lafaille; and Caitlin Anderson

1998 Staff at Alta Bates help celebrate the 101st birthday of Shie Shindo of Berkeley. Also this year: Oakland jazz musician Calvin Keys performs at a benefit for the Alta Bates Cardiac Rehab Program—10 months after he'd undergone quadruple bypass surgery at the hospital.

The Patrick T. Rankin Transplant and Apheresis Center is established as part of the Comprehensive Cancer Center at Alta Bates, and is the beneficiary of the cancer center's largest grant—a generous donation from the Rankin/Blackaller family and friends in memory of Patrick Rankin. The facility features new technology, plus music and video equipment.

(continued on page 96)

on the leading edge

Physicians have always been the common thread in the tapestry of medical excellence in the East Bay. From their very beginnings, the hospitals that now comprise Alta Bates Summit Medical Center have attracted and retained some of the Bay Area's most respected physicians. These expert, caring physicians have been innovators, teachers, researchers, and leaders who partnered with the hospitals to provide a breadth of

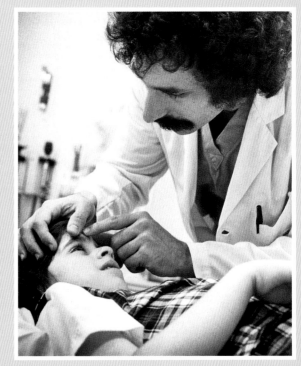

Emergency physician Stephen Schrager, MD, tends to Laiya Ghazzagh, Alta Bates, 1983.

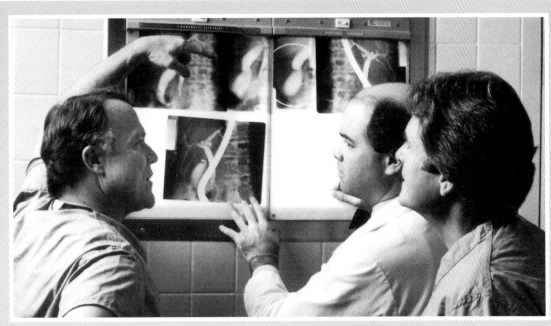

Alta Bates Drs. Charles Jenkins, N. Marcus Thygeson and Robert Fowler consult on a new laparoscopic technique to treat gallstones, 1990.

service uncommon in a community hospital.

In 1917, Frederick M. Loomis, MD, established a "first" and "best" in the East Bay by bringing anesthesia to OB services at Fabiola Hospital. (Later, he became a well-regarded Peralta physician.) Today, Alta Bates Summit doctors continue this tradition of firsts and bests with state-of-the-art procedures in heart and cancer care, minimally invasive surgery (including robotic surgery), neonatal care, and diagnostics.

As graduates of some of the most prestigious universities in the country, many members of our medical staffs have also served as associate professors at nearby prominent medical schools, sharing their expertise with young doctors. Our physicians have always had close ties with the University of California and Stanford University; their proximity is one of the reasons that our hospitals attract and retain unusually qualified physicians. At

one time, Alta Bates, Herrick, Merritt, Peralta, and Providence hospitals each had an intern and resident program in surgical and medical specialties as well as primary care. In 2004, recruitment efforts continue to attract newly trained physicians skilled in leading-edge practices.

Physicians have been valued leaders and an integral part of hospital governance since the modest beginnings of each of the five historic hospitals that constitute Alta Bates Summit. They have committed themselves to patients and communities by serving honorably on boards of trustees and as directors. This dedication to service has brought a sensitivity to diversity and the clinical requirements of quality patient care; it has also meant that the innovations of recently trained doctors are welcomed.

Throughout the years, many members of the medical staffs have been

recognized, locally and nationally, as among the best in a variety of fields. In 2004, Alta Bates Summit's 1,400 physicians are committed to community care, research, and expert innovation. More than 90 percent are board-certified in more than 50 specialties. In addition, our physicians are involved in more than 130 research studies. With such demonstrated competence and experience, our doctors are known for the exceptional quality of their diagnosis, treatment, and compassion—accomplishments that future generations of their peers are sure to uphold.

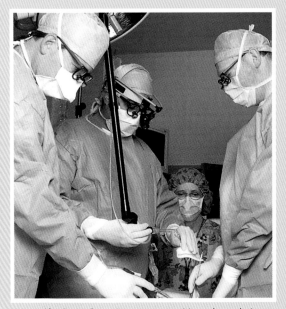

Alta Bates Summit surgeons position a laser during a state-of-the-art cardiac procedure, 2003.

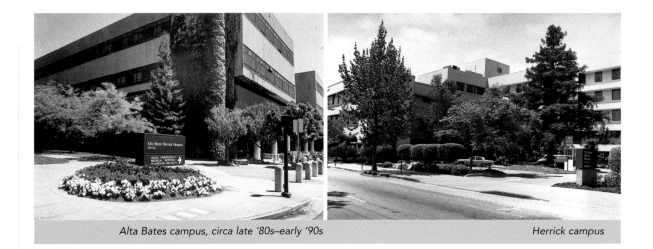

Alta Bates campus, circa late '80s–early '90s   Herrick campus

1998 As one of the first of its kind in the country, the state-of-the-art Wayne and Gladys Valley Newborn Intensive Care Unit (NICU) opens on the Alta Bates campus. The $7 million, 55-bed NICU cares for premature and sick infants in semi-private rooms in a family-friendly nursery setting. It is made possible, in large part, by the generosity of East Bay residents, particularly the Wayne and Gladys Valley Foundation, the Transamerica Foundation, and Berkeley Farms.

1998 Summit is one of only a few hospitals nationwide to participate in a Phase I clinical protocol for cardiac resynchronization therapy.

1999 Alta Bates' Respiratory Support Unit, the only hospital-based sub-acute unit of its kind in Northern California, expands from 29 to 59 beds. Hospital units for these ventilator-dependent patients are becoming increasingly difficult to find. Alta Bates is now the designated facility for the seven-county area.

1999 The Jackson Arthritis Center, dedicated to treatment of people who suffer from arthritis and related conditions, opens at Summit. The center is named for William Jackson, MD, who performed the East Bay's first total hip–replacement at Merritt in 1968, and is recognized as one of the nation's foremost experts in total joint–replacement surgery.

1999 Jerry Brown, three-time Presidential candidate and former California governor, becomes Oakland's 47th mayor.

1999 HISTORIC MERGER JOINS EAST BAY'S LEADING HOSPITALS. The December merger joins Alta Bates and Summit. The new mission statement builds on each institution's proud traditions and their vision for the future: "We enhance the health and well-being of people in

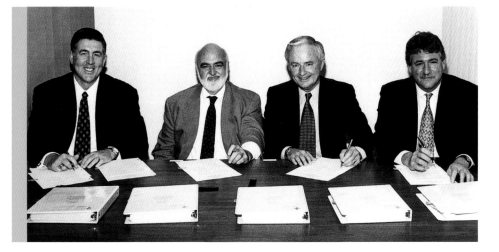

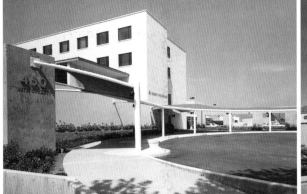

Top row, left to right: Peralta Pavilion,
Providence Pavilion, and Merritt Pavilion
Bottom row, left to right: Peralta Medical Building,
Providence Medical Building

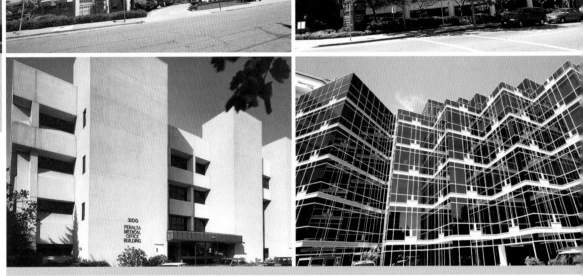

the communities we serve through compassion and excellence."

Alta Bates Summit Medical Center is an affiliate of Sutter Health, one of the nation's leading not-for-profit health care systems. Sutter Health has care centers in more than 100 Northern California communities: 26 acute-care hospitals; region-wide home health hospice and occupational health networks; and long-term care centers. Sutter has relationships with approximately 5,000 physicians.

2000 When Kaiser Permanente expands their regional cardiac service, they choose the Summit Campus of Alta Bates Summit as their new location in the East Bay.

2000 The Alta Bates Comprehensive Cancer Center celebrates its 10th year of success in patient care. At year's end, a $5,000 grant is awarded to Alta Bates Summit's Albert and Bertha Markstein Cancer Education and Prevention Center, which was named in honor of two major donors to Summit.

2000 The Alta Bates Summit Associates celebrate its 25th anniversary, continuing to operate "The Showcase—the Tiffany's of Thrift Stores" on College Avenue.

2000–2001 DOTCOM BUBBLE BURSTS.

Crashing share prices halt the speculative frenzy of investment in Internet and Internet-related technology stocks. The Bay Area, once the haven of dotcom aspirations, witnesses the demise of many companies and droves of suddenly jobless tech workers.

2001–2002 Alta Bates Summit's Ethnic Health Institute (EHI) receives $1.4 million in grants to fight prostate cancer and asthma, and to assist African Americans in end-of-life care and planning.

*facts and figures
2003*
*ALTA BATES SUMMIT
MEDICAL CENTER*

Licensed Beds: 1,082
Active Physicians: 1,679
Employees: 5,013
Volunteers: 488

alta bates summit medical center

2003 Distinguished Hospital for Clinical Excellence
—Health Grades

A Center of Expertise
—Blue Cross

Three-year accreditation for Alta Bates Blood and Marrow Transplantation Program—
one of only two Northern California medical centers to be accredited
—Foundation for the Accreditation of Cellular Therapies

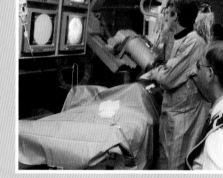

Alta Bates Summit cardiac catheterization lab

Better than Expected Outcomes in Cardiac Surgery (one of only five California hospitals)
—OSHPD and Pacific Business Group on Health

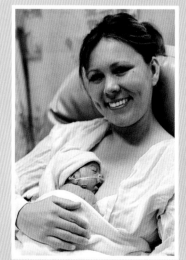

Another special delivery, 2004

Full accreditation of Rehabilitation Services
—Commission for Accreditation of Rehabilitation Facilities (CARF)

Best of the Best Birthing Center and Hospital in the East Bay
—Bay Area Parent newspaper

Best Hospital in the East Bay
—Oakland Tribune Reader's Poll

A Top 100 ICU
—Solucient (2000)

Environmental Leadership and Champions for Change Award
—Hospitals for a Healthy Environment

2001 Elena Griffing, an employee at the Alta Bates DeNicolai Burn Center, marks 49 years without a sick day at Alta Bates Hospital. In her 55-year career as an office manager and laboratory assistant, Griffing, 75, missed a total of three work days. In July 2002, Griffing becomes the last employee on the Alta Bates staff to have worked with the hospital's founder, Alta Bates.

2001 Warren J. Kirk is named President and CEO of Alta Bates Summit Medical Center, following Irwin Hansen's resignation from the post.

2001 A fundraising campaign in memory of beloved internist E. Gale Whiting Jr., MD, raises $2.1 million. In the following year, the Whiting Nuclear Medicine Center is dedicated at the Alta Bates Campus.

2002 Thunder Road, a recovery community in Oakland for youth and families struggling with substance-abuse problems, celebrates its 10th

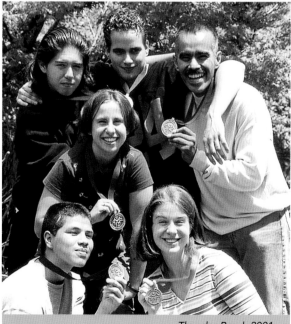

Thunder Road, 2001

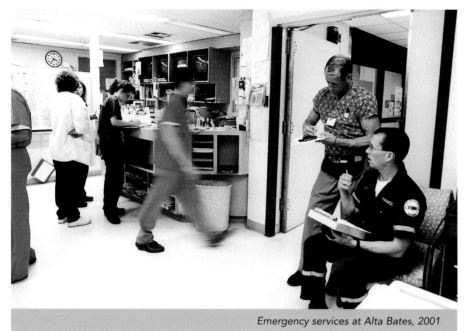
Emergency services at Alta Bates, 2001

accuracy and precision promises to speed recovery and reduce risks of complications.

2003 Alta Bates Summit Medical Center is one of the first hospitals in Northern California to use a unique "co-bedding" program in which premature twins and triplets are bedded together to promote their growth and development.

2003 Sutter Health creates a $4 million scholarship program, Sutter Scholars, benefitting the children of employees of Sutter Health affiliates.

2003 The medical center launches its new website, *www.altabatessummit.org.*

2003 Five Centers of Excellence for comprehensive health care are established at Alta Bates Summit. These specialized services, highly trained staff, and sophisticated equipment support regional tertiary programs, including Women and Infants, Cardiovascular, Minimally Invasive Surgery, Orthopedic, and Oncology Services.

2003 Alta Bates Summit Medical Center contributes more that $81 million in community benefits. It serves more than 285,000 community members through outreach services provided by the Breast Health Access for Women with Disabilities, the Ethnic Health Institute, the Health Ministry/Parish Nurse Program, Tele-Care, East Bay AIDS Center, and the Markstein Cancer Education and Prevention Center.

anniversary. The well-regarded program operates the only chemical dependency recovery hospital for youth in California.

2002 Baby Louie celebrates his second birthday in February. Louie was a micropreemie born four months early (at only 24 weeks of gestation) at Alta Bates—"hardly bigger than a pound of butter," according to press reports. The *San Francisco Chronicle* details Louie's first seven months spent in Alta Bates' NICU.

2003 ROBOTICS GO ONLINE. Alta Bates Summit's new da Vinci Surgical System (the first in Oakland and Berkeley) represents the next great wave in surgical technology and minimally invasive procedures. This technological marvel is funded, in large part, through contributions to the Foundation.

When the system is online, a surgeon sits at a video monitor a few feet away from the patient and manipulates a robotic arm that deftly controls surgical instruments. The equipment's pinpoint

facts and figures 2003
ALTA BATES SUMMIT
MEDICAL CENTER

Medicare: 32.0%

Medi-Cal: 27.5%

HMO: 22.6%

PPO: 11.7%

Other: 6.1%

THE WAY WE ARE

2000–2004:

U.S. population (2004): 294,018,772

Berkeley population (2000): 102,743

Oakland population (2000): 399,484

Life expectancy: male, 74.1; female, 79.5

Average salary (2002): $36,764

Divorce rate (2003): 3.7/1000

Viewable web pages (2004): 800 million

U.S. population that owns a cell phone (2003): 51 percent

Milk: $4.71/gallon, Bay Area; $3.66/gallon, U.S.

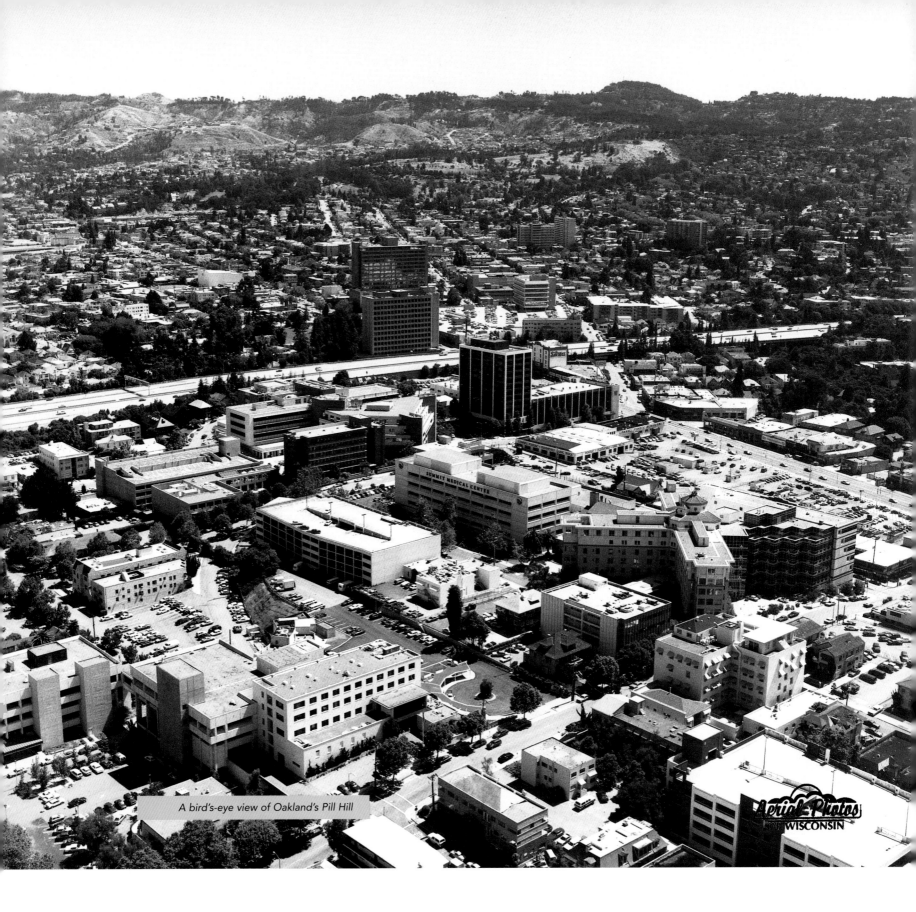

A bird's-eye view of Oakland's Pill Hill

SUMMIT MEDICAL CENTER

Aerial Photos
WISCONSIN

2003 Alta Bates Summit cardiac surgeon Junaid Khan, MD, performs the East Bay's first port access (minimally invasive) mitral valve repair.

2003 Alta Bates Summit Foundation raises a record $11.6 million in philanthropic funds, making it one of California's top community hospital foundations.

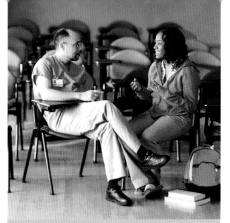

Jan Anderson confers with Youth Bridge student Krystle Thorpe, 2002.

2003 An estimated 45 million Americans are without health insurance—a record high. The percentage of uninsured increases to 15.6 percent.

2004 The campaign for the new Carol Ann Read Breast Center concludes with $2.2 million raised and a new vision for women's health in the East Bay. The Center will provide many services, with initial emphasis on expedited diagnosis of suspicious test results.

2004 Alta Bates Summit Medical Center's Blood and Marrow Transplant Program, Northern California's first, celebrates its 20th anniversary. Since its inception, more than 500 patients and their families have availed themselves of this lifesaving service.

2004 The new Women's Heart Advantage program debuts with an informative lecture series and community outreach. In concurrent presentations to doctors and nurses, the program addresses the problem of undetected and untreated heart disease in women.

2004 Alta Bates Summit Foundation launches the Centennial Campaign for Excellence, which aims to raise $25 million to help fund the hospital's new

Cardiovascular, Oncology, and Women and Infants Centers for Excellence plus five of its ongoing community programs—the East Bay AIDS Center, Ethnic Health Institute, MPI Chemical Dependency Treatment Services, The Stroke Center, and Thunder Road.

2004 Significant facilities changes pave the way for further development of clinical Centers of Excellence. Maternity services move from Summit to Alta Bates where facilities are renovated to provide more private rooms and a resource center for patients and families. Cardiovascular services expand throughout the third floor of the Merritt Pavilion, and include a resource center as well.

2005 CENTENNIAL CELEBRATION KICKS OFF A year-long calendar of events is scheduled to recognize the centennial anniversary of the founding of Alta Bates, Herrick, Merritt, Peralta, and Providence hospitals. The "Century of Caring" celebration involves employees, medical staff, volunteers, board members, and the entire community in recognizing the vast contributions of all the heritage organizations that came together as Alta Bates Summit Medical Center.

A few members of Alta Bates Summit's outstanding cardiac surgery team (clockwise from back left): Diane Brophy, RN; Coyness Ennix, MD; Annelies McNair, RN; Junaid Khan, MD; Russell Stanton, MD; Leigh Iverson, MD; and Myrna Najar, RN, 2003

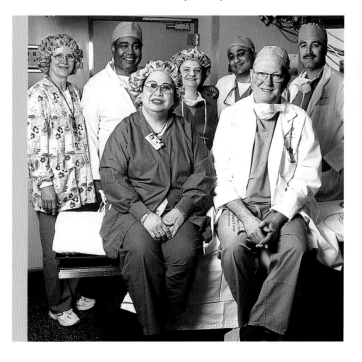

toward new frontiers

At the turn of the 21st century, a new generation of families look to Alta Bates Summit Medical Center for their care—and as our founders before us, we will be here to serve.

Health care has been and remains an awe-inspiring endeavor. Just over the horizon are exhilarating advances for the care of our patients—exciting progress in research, technological breakthroughs, advanced drug therapies—that will provide curative treatment for the most vulnerable among us. A hundred years ago, a young nurse named Alta Bates could never have imagined the lifesaving procedures and devices used today in the care of tiny premature infants in our Newborn Intensive Care Unit. And the promise of tomorrow holds even more astounding opportunities to provide care.

Major medical advances will lead us to more effective use for robotic surgery, to gene therapy for many now incurable diseases, and to bypass surgery without the use of sutures. Stem cell therapy, genomics, minimally invasive surgery to treat any

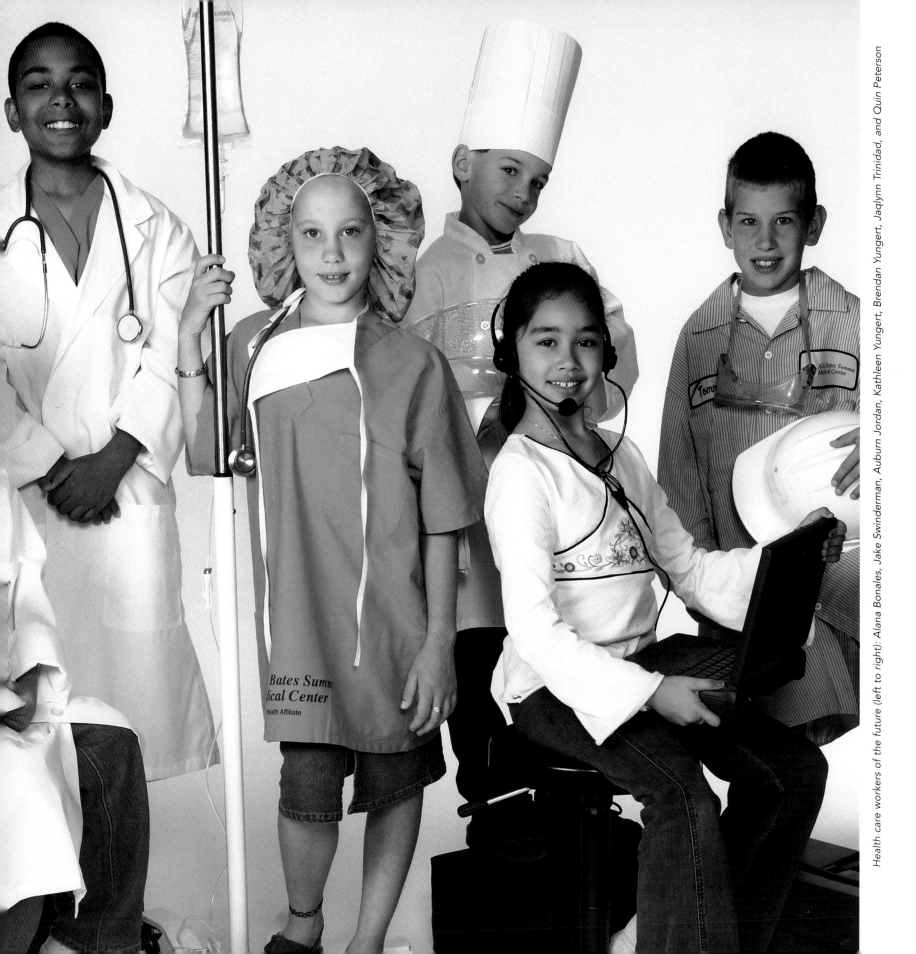

part of the body, and improved techniques in risk assessment, diagnosis, and treatment of cancer patients only hint at what awaits us. Imagine the miracles the future holds for our families.

As medical breakthroughs and advances expand our ability to heal, we also achieve better and broader ways of reaching out to our diverse communities, and we have great confidence in our ability to close gaps in health care access and delivery. Though available resources are strained, the Medical Center remains committed to leading the way in addressing health needs that ultimately impact us all.

To ensure the next century of caring, the Alta Bates Summit Foundation has launched the Centennial Campaign for Excellence, the most significant community-wide fundraising effort ever mounted on behalf of East Bay health care. With an ambitious goal of raising $25 million, the Centennial Campaign for Excellence will fund needed expansion in the areas of Cardiology, Oncology, and Women and Infants as well as community benefit programs that target other areas of concern, including chemical dependency and health disparities.

Throughout its 100-year history, Alta Bates Summit Medical Center has maintained a proud tradition of service to the community partnered with philanthropy. The generosity of community members who have helped us to bring excellence in health care to all who live here is legendary.

Now, as we begin our second hundred years, a new team of physicians, staff, and enthusiastic volunteers leads us. As we continue striving for excellence in patient care, we embark on a new era of safeguarding and fostering good health in those we serve. Most important, our commitment to expand and enhance programs gives our community the security that, whatever comes their way, Alta Bates Summit Medical Center will be here to care for them.

In many ways, Alta Bates Summit is the heart of this region. Our children are born here, and generations of families have turned to us for care. Improving the health of our community has been, and will remain, the medical center's mission. We look forward to caring for generations to come.

■ ■ ■

boards of trustees and administrative leaders

1903–2004

ALTA BATES SUMMIT MEDICAL CENTER BOARD OF TRUSTEES CHAIRS

Mary Brown
Lawrence D. Fox

ALTA BATES SUMMIT MEDICAL CENTER ADMINISTRATIVE LEADERS

Warren J. Kirk
Irwin Hansen

SUMMIT MEDICAL CENTER BOARD OF TRUSTEES CHAIRS

James D. Falaschi

SUMMIT MEDICAL CENTER ADMINISTRATIVE LEADERS

Irwin Hansen
Kenneth M. Jones

ALTA BATES HERRICK AND ALTA BATES MEDICAL CENTER BOARD OF TRUSTEES CHAIRS

Carol D'Onofrio, DrPH
Alan Lifshay, MD
David L. Cutter
Richard L. Oken, MD

ALTA BATES HERRICK AND ALTA BATES MEDICAL CENTER ADMINISTRATIVE LEADERS

Alan Lifshay, MD
George Caralis
Albert L. Greene
Paul Hoffman
Eleanor G. Claus, RN, MSN

ALTA BATES CORPORATION BOARD OF TRUSTEES CHAIRS

Steven H. Oliver
Robert S. Manlove

ALTA BATES CORPORATION ADMINISTRATIVE LEADERS

Robert L. Montgomery*
Kenneth W. Sargent
Byron Irwin
Robert L. Montgomery*

MERRITT PERALTA BOARD OF TRUSTEES CHAIRS

James D. Falaschi
William F. Ausfahl
George C. Hill
Gordon Huber, Jr.
Steven V. White
Wayne E. Thompson
C. Lee Emerson

MERRITT PERALTA ADMINISTRATIVE LEADERS

Kenneth M. Jones
Lee Domanico
Richard J. McCann

ALTA BATES BOARD OF TRUSTEES CHAIRS

Steven H. Oliver
Henrik L. Blum, MD
Robert G. Eaneman
Robert S. Manlove
Stephen L. Davenport
Alvin W. Langfield
Raymond M. Young
Laverne H. Kibbe
E.C. Pitcher
Alta Alice Miner Bates, RN

ALTA BATES ADMINISTRATIVE LEADERS

Eleanor G. Claus, RN, MSN
Kenneth W. Sargent
David D. O'Neill
Robert L. Montgomery
John E. Peterson
James Voss
John A. Wentworth
Alta Alice Miner Bates, RN

HERRICK BOARD OF TRUSTEES CHAIRS

Suren H. Babington, MD
Wanda H. Stanley
Leland H. Cohn, MD
Ivadell Herrick Henderson

HERRICK ADMINISTRATIVE LEADERS

John Martin
Gary Pasama
Hershel W. Shelton
John F. Wight
Alfred E. Maffly
LeRoy Francis Herrick, MD

MERRITT BOARD OF TRUSTEES CHAIRS

Laine J. Ainsworth
Marshall Steel, Jr.
Lawrence S. Simon
Gordon H. Huber

MERRITT ADMINISTRATIVE LEADERS

Richard J. McCann
Richard Wickel
Richard Highsmith
Harrison Rowe

PERALTA BOARD OF TRUSTEES

C. Lee Emerson
A. G. Thies
Bert Railey

PERALTA ADMINISTRATIVE LEADERS

Robert S. Mason
George U. Wood, PharmD

PROVIDENCE COMMUNITY ADVISORY BOARD CHAIRS

Sister Karin Dufault
John P. Ablan
John Sparrow
William Stephens
Ray Rinehart
Terrence Y. LaCroix
John L. McDonnell
Glenn Malley, MD
James E. Roberts
Robert C. Burnstein
Sister Lucille Dean

PROVIDENCE ADMINISTRATIVE LEADERS

David D. O'Neill
Sister Dona Taylor
W. Stewart Tittle
Peter Bigelow
Stanley W. Volga
Sister Francis Ignatius (Gladys Teresa MacDowell)
Sister Charles Raymond (Therese Yvette Bilodeau)
Sister Yves of Providence (Yvette Lalonde)
Sister Bonosa (Elizabeth Marshall)
Sister Peter Francis* (Zelie Bourdage)
Sister Anne Philomena (Rose Alba Latour)
Sister Peter Francis* (Zelie Bourdage)
Sister Joseph Ignatius (Ernestine Quenneville)
Sister Gertrude of Providence (Clara Ann O'Brien)
Sister Angelica (Ellen Elizabeth MacKinnon)
Sister Mary Alice (Margaret Catherine Woods)
Sister Mary of Nazareth (Catherine O'Donnell)
Sister Joseph Albert (Amanda Jutras)
Mother Mary Theresa (M. Rosalia Muller)

* Two terms of service

sources

In the creation of *A Century of Caring*, the primary sources of information were published historial accounts and Alta Bates Summit Medical Center and its five historic hospitals' 100-year collection of archival materials, including historical photographs, hospital literature, exhibits, and other artifacts. The institutions' publications were especially helpful, including: Alta Bates Hospital's 75th Anniversary Publication; *Alta Bates News*; *Community Connection; Herrick Hospitaler; Merritt Monogram; The Peraltan; Partners in Care;* and *Providence Hospital of Oakland: 1904-1992, 88 Years of History.*

OTHER PRINT SOURCES
Asian Week, "APA History Timeline." May 2004.
Bagwell, Elizabeth. *Oakland: The Story of a City.* Novato, CA: Presidio Press, 1982.
Berkeley Daily Gazette: February 20, May 8 and 9, August 6 and 9, December 20, 1945; December 1, 1955; February 19, 1957; June 19, 1968.
Butler, Mary Ellen. *Oakland Welcomes the World.* Montgomery, AL: Community Communications Inc., 1996.
Caldwell, Bill. *Oakland: A Photographic Journey.* Oakland: Momentum Publications, 2003.
Fibel, Pearl Randolph. *The Peraltas.* Oakland: Peralta Hospital, 1971.
Garrison, F. *Introduction to the History of Medicine.* Philadelphia: WB Saunders, Co., 1913.
HandPrints, "Children's Hospital Oakland Celebrates Its 90th Birthday." Fall 2002.
"Henry J. Kaiser Think Big," January 24–August 29, 2004 exhibition shown at the Oakland Museum of California.

Hill, Kimi Kodani, ed. *Shades of California.* Berkeley, CA: Heyday Books, 2001.
Koford, Henning, MD. *Dr. Samuel Merritt— His Life and Achievements.* n.p.: Oakland, 1938.
Lemke, Gretchen. "Afro Americans in Berkeley, 1859-1987" (monograph).
LeMone, Priscilla, Carol Lillis and Carol Taylor. *Fundamentals of Nursing.* Philadelphia: J.B. Lippincott Company, 1993.
Looking Back at Berkeley. Berkeley, CA: Berkeley History Book Committee of the Berkeley Historical Society, 1984.
Marion, Lucy, PhD, RN, CS. *Nursing's Vision for Primary Health Care in the 21st Century.* Washington, D. C.: American Nurses Association, 1996.
Perry, Anne Griffin and Patricia A. Potter. *Basic Nursing.* St. Louis: Mosby, 1999.
Reed, Ishmael. *Blues City.* New York: Crown Journeys, 2003.
Saragoza, Alex. *Life Stories: Voices From the East Bay Latino Community.* Oakland: Oakland Museum of California, 2003.
Schwartz, Richard. *Berkeley 1900: Daily Life at the Turn of the Century.* n.p.: RSB Books, 2000.
Sebastian, Anton. *Dates in Medicine: A Chronological Record of Medical Progress Over Three Millennia.* New York: CRC Press–Parthenon Publishers, 2000.
Shutes, Milton Henry, MD. *A History of the Alameda County Medical Association.* Berkeley, CA: The Howell North Press, 1947.
Snodgrass, Mary Ellen. *Historical Encyclopedia of Nursing.* Santa Barbara, CA: ABC-CLIO, 1999.
Trager, James. *The People's Chronology: A Year-by-Year Record of Human Events From Prehistory to the Present.* Orlando, FL: Harcourt School Publications, 1979.
Wasserman, Abby, ed. *The Spirit of Oakland: An Anthology.* Oakland:

Heritage Media Corporation, 2000.
Wetterau, Bruce. *New York Public Library Book of Chronologies.* New York: Macmillian General Reference, 1990.

INTERNET SOURCES
Berkeley Public Library Online, http://berkeleypubliclibrary.org
City of Oakland Centennial Timeline, http://www.oaklandnet.com
Doctor Spock Company Online, http://www.drspock.com
Encyclopaedia Britannica Online, http://www.britannica.com
Free Speech Movement Archives Online http://www.fsm-a.org
California History Online, http://www.californiahistory.net
National Asian American Telecommunications Association Online, http://www.naatanet.org
National Women's Health Information Center Online, http://www.4woman.gov
Nobel Prize E-Museum, http://nobelprize.org
Oakland Museum of California, http://collections.museumca.org
Park Net–The National Park Service Online, http://www.nps.gov
United Nations Online, http://www.un.org
Wollenberg, Charles. *Berkeley, a City History,* http://www.infopeople.org/bpl/system/historytext.html.

PHOTO CREDITS
Courtesy African American Museum and Library at Oakland (AAMLO), 25, 28, 45.
Courtesy The Bancroft Library, University of California, Berkeley, 41 (10035258A), 48 (j14GA-542B), 69 (00040908b_c), 70 (10007446A).
Courtesy Berkeley Historical Society, 39 (#4.5.3.193), 60 (#1.1.4.195.0626),